Heart
Trouble
Encyclopedia

Heart Trouble Encyclopedia

M. Gabriel Khan, M.D.
Henry J. L. Marriott, M.D.

Published in 1996 by
Stoddart Publishing Co. Limited
34 Lesmill Road
Toronto, Canada M3B 2T6
Tel. (416) 445-3333
Fax (416) 445-5967

Stoddart Books are available for bulk purchase for
sales promotions, premiums, fundraising, and seminars. For details,
contact the **Special Sales Department** at the above address.

Canadian Cataloguing in Publication Data

Khan, M. Gabriel
Heart trouble encyclopedia

ISBN 0-7737-5744-9

1. Heart – Disease – Popular works.

I. Marriott, Henry J. L. (Henry Joseph Llewellyn), 1917– .
II. Title.

RC681.K53 1995   616.1'2   C95-931222-6

Cover Design: the boy 100 & Tannice Goddard
Computer Layout: Tannice Goddard
Printed and bound in Canada

*The author and the publisher cannot be held responsible for damages
incurred by patients in using the information given in this book,
be it related to nondrug or drug treatment.
Patients are strongly advised to follow the directives of their doctor at all times.
The information given in this book is to be used
only along with the advice of your doctor.*

Contents

PREFACE

In producing *Heart Trouble Encyclopedia*, our aim has been to provide readers with an accurate and up-to-date book that covers all aspects of heart ailments. Heart disease, including high blood pressure, affects more than 70 million individuals in North America and is the leading cause of death, stroke and disability in North America, Europe, the United Kingdom and Russia.

Fortunately, recent major medical breakthroughs have brought hope to many. This book presents readers with information on these life-saving treatments and other recognized methods of therapy currently available. Chest pain is the commonest complaint of a patient suffering from heart trouble; this text gives the reader a clear description of the many causes of chest pain, including pain caused by angina or a heart attack.

We believe that our title, *Heart Trouble Encyclopedia*, is appropriate. The *Oxford Dictionary* defines an encyclopedia as a work containing information on some one art or branch of knowledge arranged systematically. Our book gives an accurate, comprehensive and systematic account of all common heart ailments with their nondrug and drug therapies.

There are several books available on heart diseases; why then another book? Many of the books that have been available during the past 20 years are anecdotal. They give treatment schedules, dietary recipes and programs that originate from the author's concepts, and are not based on current scientific literature. There are books that give advice on how to cure a cholesterol problem in eight weeks, an unbelievable and impossible feat! There are books that claim the cure of heart disease by diets, meditation and special exercises. The hopeful reader is dismayed finally by the false reports and anecdotal accounts. Available books may discuss the cholesterol problem and heart attacks, but do not cover other heart problems, particularly in-depth accounts of how to cope with angina, high blood pressure, heart murmurs, diseased heart valves, heart failure, heart muscle disease and pericarditis.

We feel a complete work should be a valuable household asset for family reference. There has been much talk recently concerning aspirin, estrogens, vitamin E, beta-carotene, other antioxidants and women and heart disease; these topics are given accurate coverage in our book. The bibliography provided at the back of the text gives a list of articles that pertain to clinical studies described in the book.

The statistics citing the incidence of cardiovascular disease are derived from the United States, particularly the National Center for Health Statistics. The incidence of cardiovascular disease in Canada is approximately 10 percent of the figures given for the United States.

We are certain that readers will not be dismayed or lose faith in our written material. The treatment schedules are not ours, but are derived from a thorough review of the world scientific literature on nondrug and drug management of heart diseases. The regimens have been approved by consensus panels of the American Heart Association and other national committees. We must emphasize, however, that you should use the information in this book along with the advice of your doctor.

Lastly, we must commend the efforts of Donald Bastian and Kevin Linder of Stoddart Publishing and the invaluable secretarial assistance of Hazel Luce and Lynne Rose.

ANEURYSM

An aneurysm is a ballooning of the wall of an artery or the heart caused by severe weakening of the walls of the artery or the heart muscle.

The largest artery in the body is the aorta, which takes blood from the heart and runs from the chest into the abdomen, lying against the spine until it reaches the pelvis, dividing at that point into iliac arteries that supply blood to the pelvis, buttocks and legs (see Fig. 4). Because the aorta takes the full force of blood ejected from the heart, it is the commonest artery in the body to weaken. This artery is also commonly affected by the process of atherosclerosis (see Atherosclerosis). The elastic wall of the aorta may be stretched and weakened, especially in the abdomen. Most aneurysms occur in the abdomen just after the aorta branches to the kidney and before the aorta ends in its division into iliac arteries to the pelvis (see Fig. 4). The normal diameter of the aorta is 1.8 to 2 cm. Aneurysms are significant when they are greater than 4 cm in diameter. Other sites for aneurysm formation are in the thoracic aorta, the iliac arteries in the pelvis and the popliteal artery at the back of the knee.

Weakening of arteries occurs because of atherosclerosis and loss of elasticity due to aging; high blood pressure increases the process of aneurysm formation and rupture. Patients with Marfan's syndrome, a disease that affects the elasticity of arterial walls, may develop aneurysms. Studies indicate that there is a familial incidence of abdominal aortic aneurysms.

The occurrence of aneurysms is not uncommon in men over age 60. Aneurysms may grow to more than 5 cm without causing symptoms and may go unnoticed by the individual. A simple ultrasound of the abdomen detects all abdominal aneurysms and gives a good estimate of their size.

TREATMENT

Major surgery is indicated when aneurysms are greater than 5 or 6 cm. Recently, stents have been used successfully to reinforce the artery wall. This technique involves minor surgery. A stent, a tube of variable length made of stainless steel or other material, is introduced through an artery in the leg and is advanced to the area of weakness in the artery. The stent serves as an inner lining that strengthens the artery wall. This represents a major break-through because many patients with aneurysms are elderly and have other diseases, particularly prior heart attacks, which carry an increased risk for major surgical intervention.

Berry Aneurysm

A different type of aneurysm may occur at the base of the brain. The arteries at this site may have a developmental defect and form small berry-like aneurysms that may remain asymptomatic until a rupture occurs when the individual is between 20 and 50 years old. Bleeding, or subarachnoid hemorrhage, at the base of the brain may damage the brain substance. These aneurysms may cause sudden intense headaches. Fortunately, these aneurysms can be clipped off prior to their rupture. Berry aneurysms are not related to high blood pressure, but coexisting hypertension may predispose them to rupture. Patients with coarctation or polycystic kidneys may have coexisting berry aneurysms.

ANGINA

Pain or discomfort in the chest, throat, jaw or arms caused by severe, but temporary, lack of blood and oxygen to a part of the heart muscle (see Fig. 1).

Angina affects more than 40 million North Americans. The treatment of angina, which includes coronary angioplasty and coronary bypass surgery, costs more than $40 billion annually in the United States. Angina causes suffering, disability and financial

CORONARY HEART (ARTERY) DISEASE

FIGURE 1

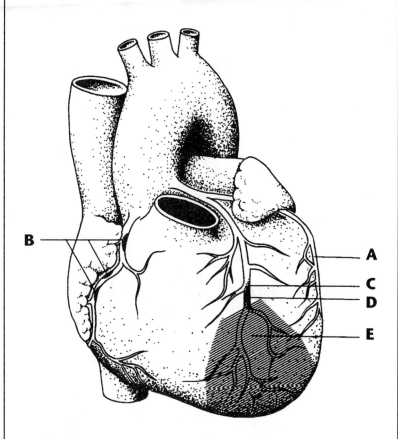

A Normal coronary artery
B Obstruction of a coronary artery by atherosclerosis causing less blood to reach the heart muscle, producing chest pain, called angina
C Blood clot
D Complete obstruction of a coronary artery by atherosclerosis and blood clot (coronary thrombosis), causing E
E Damage and death of heart muscle cells, i.e., a heart attack (myocardial infarction)

CORONARY ARTERIES

FIGURE 2

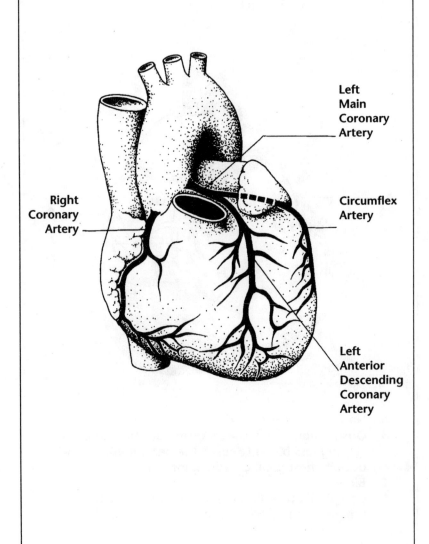

Left
Main
Coronary
Artery

Circumflex
Artery

Right
Coronary
Artery

Left
Anterior
Descending
Coronary
Artery

hardship. Angina affects men more commonly than women, and the underlying disease condition is not surprisingly referred to as "the widow-maker."

CAUSES

A high blood cholesterol, and other factors along with a genetic background, causes damage to arteries, finally leading to blockage, especially in the coronary arteries that feed the heart muscle with blood (see Fig. 1). The heart muscle is one of the strongest in the body and as powerful as the muscle of the thigh and legs. The act of walking or running requires contraction of the leg muscles. Such muscle work or activity requires efficient delivery of oxygen, glucose and other nutrients, which are brought from the heart to the muscles by blood vessels called arteries. The heart, our lifeline, functions as a simple pump that pumps more than 250 million liters of blood in an individual's average lifetime. *It is surprising, therefore, that the muscle of this important pump receives a supply of blood via only three small arteries that have a diameter of a soda straw, ranging from 3 to 7 mm* (see Fig. 2). The coronary arteries run along the surface of the heart and are branches of the largest artery in the body, the aorta, which commences at the left ventricle, the main pumping chamber of the heart (see Fig. 2). If the arteries that feed the heart muscle with blood become partially blocked, the muscle becomes painful when it is being used.

As far back as the time of the Caesars, pain in the legs due to obstruction of blood flow in arteries to the legs was labeled as *intermittent claudication*. The Emperor Claudius limped because of a painful leg, and the word claudication is derived from his name. Similarly, angina is the name for chest pain of short duration that originates from the heart muscle because of a reduced blood supply. The blood contains essential nutrients, particularly oxygen, that are vital to the function of the heart and all body cells.

From about age 30 onwards the coronary arteries become slowly obstructed by sludge, consisting of cholesterol and smaller blood particles called platelets. The sludge forms a hardness, or plaque, which doctors call *atheroma*. These plaques bulge into the interior of the arteries, obstructing the free flow of blood (see Figs. 1, 3). The word "atheroma" is derived from the Greek "athere" meaning porridge or gruel. When a plaque of atheroma is

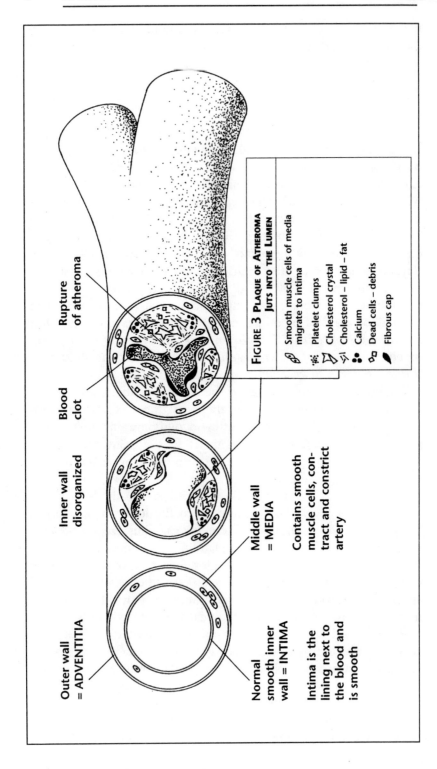

Outer wall
= ADVENTITIA

Inner wall
disorganized

Rupture
of atheroma

Blood
clot

Normal
smooth inner
wall = INTIMA

Intima is the
lining next to
the blood and
is smooth

Middle wall
= MEDIA

Contains smooth
muscle cells, con-
tract and constrict
artery

FIGURE 3 PLAQUE OF ATHEROMA
JUTS INTO THE LUMEN

Smooth muscle cells of media
migrate to intima

Platelet clumps

Cholesterol crystal

Cholesterol – lipid – fat

Calcium

Dead cells – debris

Fibrous cap

cut open, one can see a gelatinous, porridge-like material which contains cholesterol. Fortunately, this porridge-like fatty material does not touch the blood that flows through the artery because nature covers the fatty material with a protective hard layer of cells called fibrous tissue. A plaque of atheroma therefore consists of a central fatty core, covered by a fibrous cap (see Fig. 3).

Fibrous tissue is formed from special cells that are produced everywhere in the body when a repair job is needed; for example, a few days after a large cut or surgical wound is stitched, fibrous tissue cells move in to form a bridge, which transforms over the next weeks into a scar. Fibrous tissue forms scars. Some scars are smooth; some are bumpy and rough. So are the plaques of atheroma sometimes smooth or bumpy and rough. These tough scars in the inner wall of the arteries are perhaps nature's way of patching and healing. Because the vessel wall affected by atheroma gets hardened and the medical word for hardness is "sclerosis," the term used for this disease is *atherosclerosis.* Plaques of atheroma are most commonly found in the abdominal aorta where it divides to form the vessels to the pelvis and lower limbs, in the coronary arteries, in the carotid arteries to the neck and brain and in the vessels of the lower limbs (see Fig. 4).

When atherosclerosis in the coronary arteries causes symptoms, doctors use the term "atherosclerotic heart disease." Many doctors use the term "ischemic heart disease" because ischemia means a lack of blood/oxygen. Others use the term "coronary heart disease," and since the latter term is more commonly used, we will use it in this book. Angina and heart attacks are the two main manifestations of coronary heart disease.

When a coronary artery is severely obstructed with plaque, the heart muscle still receives an adequate amount of oxygen when the heart is at rest and beating slowly, at about 72 beats per minute. During exertion or undue stress, however, the heart rate may increase from 72 to 90 or more beats per minute. A faster heart rate entails more work for the heart, which in turn requires more oxygen to accomplish the work. But the obstruction to the artery does not allow sufficient oxygenated blood to reach the heart muscle. During those few moments, the lack of oxygen causes the heart muscle to become painful, and this sensation is perceived by the individual as pain or merely a mild but bothersome discomfort in the chest.

Fortunately, no damage happens to the heart muscle during an attack of angina. Full recovery occurs within minutes of the attack.

HEART AND ARTERIES

FIGURE 4

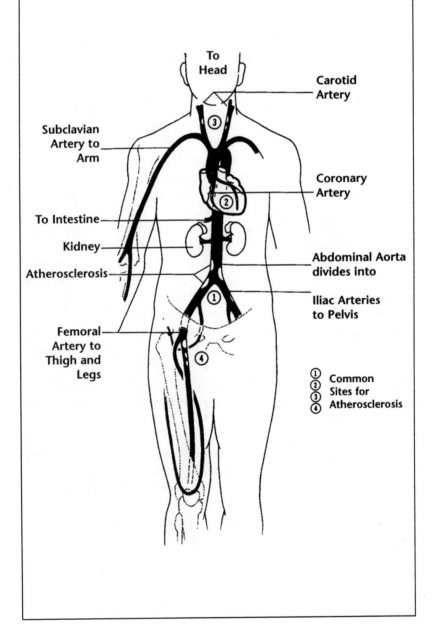

Many patients have several episodes of this fleeting pain or discomfort a few times monthly for over 15 years and learn to cope with the minor restrictions to their lifestyle. In some individuals, angina worsens and requires special therapy; some patients go on to have heart attacks.

PAIN PATTERN

The pain of angina is usually felt in the center of the chest over the breastbone, and only rarely over the breasts (see Fig. 5). Pain in the lower jaw accompanied by pain in the chest or arms during a walk or strenuous activity is nearly always due to angina, especially if these symptoms recur during similar activities. Sometimes the discomfort is only in the upper arm with a tingling feeling in

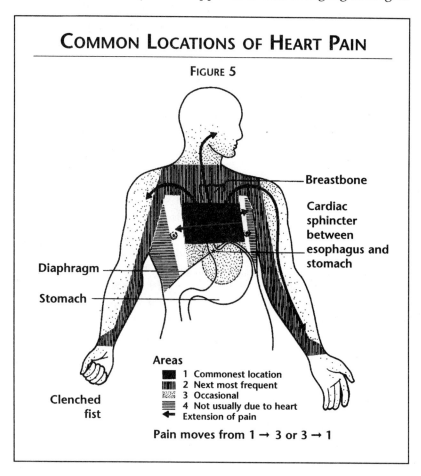

COMMON LOCATIONS OF HEART PAIN

FIGURE 5

Breastbone

Cardiac
sphincter
between
esophagus and
stomach

Diaphragm

Stomach

Clenched
fist

Areas
■ 1 Commonest location
▥ 2 Next most frequent
▦ 3 Occasional
▤ 4 Not usually due to heart
← Extension of pain

Pain moves from 1 → 3 or 3 → 1

the fingers; this pain comes mainly on exertion as opposed to pain produced, for example, by a pinched nerve. A pinched nerve will cause similar discomfort in the arms and fingers when the individual is at rest, but an activity, such as walking, makes little difference.

The pain of angina may be mild to moderate and only occasionally severe. Often it is a mere discomfort. The individual may even refuse to use the word pain to describe the peculiar sensation that feels like a tightness or a heavy weight on the breastbone. To some it's a burning sensation and to others a feeling of strangulation or suffocation that fortunately disappears within one to five minutes of rest, either with the individual standing or sitting. The pain of angina rarely lasts more than 10 minutes. If your pain is similar to that described and lasts more than 15 minutes, you should call your physician and go immediately to a hospital emergency room.

Although we have already described angina for you, the description given by William Heberden in 1768 is worth quoting. Heberden gave a detailed description of a peculiar type of chest discomfort suffered by his patients and he adopted the term "angina pectoris." His description was most appropriate:

"There is a disorder of the breasts marked with strong and peculiar symptoms, considerable for the kind of danger belonging to it, and not extremely rare which deserves to be mentioned more at length. The site of it, and the sense of strangling and anxiety with which it is attended, may make it not improperly called angina pectoris.

"They who are affected with it are seized while they are walking (more especially if it be uphill, and soon after eating) with a painful and most disagreeable sensation in the breasts, which seems as if it were to extinguish life, if it were to increase or continue; but the moment they stand still, all this uneasiness vanishes.

"In all other respects, the patients are, at the beginning of this disorder, perfectly well, and in particular have no shortness of breath, from which it is totally different. The pain is sometimes situated in the upper part, sometimes in the middle, sometimes at the bottom of the os sterni, and often more inclined to the left than to the right. It likewise very frequently extends from the breasts to the middle of the left arm."

Heberden recognized that the pain of angina always got better within a minute or so after the precipitating activity was stopped. For example, the individual might be quite well, but on walking up an incline, especially against the wind, he or she develops discomfort in the chest. If the individual stops the walk immediately and rests a minute, thus allowing the heart work to decrease, the discomfort disappears immediately.

This concept of oxygen supply versus its demand by the heart muscle is the hallmark of angina. Your doctor will ask you about your symptoms and will try to draw this information from you. You can make a long list of what precipitates the pain and what relieves it, but the one important clue to help both you and your doctor is that the pain or discomfort is precipitated by a particular activity and, once you stop the activity, the pain disappears within minutes.

Activities That Precipitate Angina

1. Walking up a hill.
2. Walking against the wind.
3. Running with some associated anxiety for a bus or to a place, especially while carrying a bag. Anxiety is made more profound if the individual is late and must rush. Thus, there is exertion and emotional stress.
4. A brisk walk or similar exertion soon after eating. This does not include bending and stooping, which can precipitate indigestion.
5. Unaccustomed exertion.
6. Emotional distress; for example, bad news, a scare, anger, rage, nightmares and the like.
7. In patients with angina, pain may occur during overwhelming excitement; for example, watching your team playing football, hockey, baseball, basketball and similar exciting programs.

STABLE AND UNSTABLE ANGINA

There are two types of angina: stable angina and unstable angina. Angina is described as stable if the condition has been present for more than two months, or if there has been no change in the pattern of pain, particularly no change in the frequency of attacks, severity or duration of pain. Patients with stable angina do not get pain at rest, except if caused by *sudden emotional stress*. Angina is described as unstable when angina is present for less than 60 days, or when there is an increase in the frequency, severity and duration of pain and a change in the known precipitating factors. If pain that normally occurs only on exertion or moderate activities starts to occur on minimal activity or at rest but *without emotional stress*, a patient should seek urgent attention in the emergency room of a hospital.

CASE HISTORY: PATIENT WITH ANGINA

A 54-year-old man was late for a job interview. With some difficulty, he found a parking space. It was a very cold and windy January day, and he walked quickly for about two hundred yards toward the building. Suddenly, he felt a strange sensation in his chest. He kept on walking, but about a minute later the discomfort felt like a heavy weight on his breastbone. His chest felt tight as he reached the building, and he rested against the wall. He took a few deep breaths and felt better after about one minute. He had his job interview without any further discomfort and remained pain-free until a few months later when, while walking up an incline, he felt a similar pain. Again he had to stop for a minute or two to get relief from the strange feeling of suffocation or strangulation that accompanied the tight feeling in his upper chest. The next day he was able to walk about a mile at a normal pace on a level grade without chest discomfort. A few days later he went golfing; during the first nine holes he felt well and had no chest discomfort. But walking the long 11th par 5, up slopes, he felt pressure in his chest, a tightness across the shoulder and a heaviness in his arms. He stopped pulling his golf cart and stood still for a minute. Somewhat embarrassed for holding up the game, he searched his golf bag for some antacid tablets but, as he opened the package, he noticed the pain had completely gone. He felt well that night. The next day when he walked quickly the discomfort returned. His wife insisted on a visit to the doctor. The doctor found him to be slightly overweight with a normal electrocardiogram reading. He was given nitroglycerin to be used under the tongue and an oral nitrate called isosorbide dinitrate in tablet form to help dilate the coronary arteries and relieve pain.

During the next three months, the man suffered from severe headaches that lasted a couple of hours after taking his medication. His chest discomfort did not get worse, but his wife insisted on a referral to a cardiologist. The cardiologist confirmed the diagnosis of stable angina and recommended that the man follow a weight-reducing, low-cholesterol, low-saturated fat diet and that he stop smoking. The cardiologist discontinued the oral nitrate drug and replaced it with timolol, a beta-blocking drug, which produced further relief of chest pain during the next year.

WEIGHT REDUCTION EFFECTS

If you have angina and you lose 10 to 25 pounds in weight, you will certainly experience less pain; you will require a smaller dose of antianginal medication, and may not require angioplasty or surgery.

Weight reduction, relief of stress, a low-saturated fat diet and avoidance of smoking are the most important nondrug treatments for patients with angina. Weight loss depends on eating less calories and burning off more calories during exercise. You must combine a low-calorie diet with some form of exercise that increases caloric expenditure, otherwise you will not be able to prevent the weight gain that often occurs six months or so after stopping a low-calorie diet. *All diets that are proven to cause weight loss over a period of years depend on reduced intake of calories.* Calories *do* count, don't let anyone tell you otherwise.

You will lose weight if you reduce your calorie intake to less than 1,000 calories daily and burn off more calories by exercise. A meal should contain a moderate amount of protein, but a low saturated fat content. Reduce your intake of high-calorie foods containing refined sugars or starches. Fish three times weekly, even canned tuna, salmon, sardine and herring, will help to reduce the saturated fat in your diet. Many individuals may stick to these rules, but forget that alcohol, both mixes and beer, are high in calories. Avoid fast foods because they often contain a lot of calories and are usually high in salt. An increase in salt increases the work of the heart muscle and puts a strain on the heart, which can lead to heart failure and shortness of breath. Thus, patients with high blood pressure, heart failure and angina are the three groups that are advised to follow a low-salt diet.

Lack of motivation often results in a failure to reduce weight. It is too tough a battle for most overweight individuals on their own, and success is more often obtained by joining a weight-loss program or clinic. We strongly advise you to consult your physician or to contact your Heart and Stroke Association for recommended publications on weight loss.

EXERCISE

Now, what about exercise and angina? An exercise stress test using a treadmill or bicycle under the supervision of your physician should provide the answer to the question, "How much exercise is safe for me?" Usually, a safe level of exercise is that which will bring on only mild discomfort or mild shortness of breath. You should slow down for a few seconds then stop for a minute or so before continuing the activity (such as a further quarter or half-mile walk). Stretching exercises and walking — including climbing two or three flights of stairs daily — will improve your muscle tone. Exercise alone, however, cannot remove the obstruction caused by plaques in arteries. Patients with angina do not jog because this activity often precipitates pain.

SMOKING

Nonsmoking men are 10 times less likely to have a fatal or nonfatal heart attack than heavy smokers. Sudden death by heart attack is more common in heavy smokers than in nonsmokers. Drugs that are effective in preventing angina and death lose their effectiveness in smokers because the by-products of cigarettes interfere with the drugs in the liver; also, grafts become blocked within a few years of bypass surgery in patients who continue to smoke. If you have angina and chronic bronchitis, cigarette smoking will cause an increase in shortness of breath.

Women between the ages of 35 and 50 who have functioning ovaries rarely suffer from angina or have heart attacks. Women who smoke and have an elevated blood cholesterol level, unfortunately, increase their risk of having a heart attack, angina or stroke.

Perhaps, rather than quitting, you have considered changing to a different brand of cigarettes. The bad news is that filter cigarettes, low-nicotine or low-tar brands of cigarettes do not decrease the risk of heart attacks. In fact, filter cigarettes deliver more carbon monoxide to the smoker's system and cause more heart attacks than do plain cigarettes. Carbon monoxide is a dangerous component of cigarette smoking.

The oxygen supply to the heart muscle is low in patients with angina. We know that angina patients who are smokers experience pain at lower levels of exercise. Nicotine causes a slight increase in the heart rate and a rise in blood pressure; therefore, the heart muscle demands more oxygen. Carbon monoxide steals oxygen away from the heart muscle, which is already deprived of oxygen. So the combination of carbon monoxide and nicotine is bad news. Regardless of the present condition of your heart, you can do yourself no greater favor than to quit smoking.

Still, how do you stop smoking? We all know that it is easier said than done. The first step is motivation.

Consider the facts. The dangers of carbon monoxide are well known. You wouldn't stand around inhaling exhaust fumes from a car, especially if its engine was running in an enclosed garage; you know that that situation would cause death. Yet, we have information today that proves heavy cigarette smokers are exposed to *eight times* the level of carbon monoxide considered safe in industry, and it has been proven that heavy cigarette smoking is a cause of heart attacks and sudden death.

The addiction of nicotine is so powerful that our words and those of others will not suffice if the motivation is not there. You will note that we have not lectured on cigarette smoking as a cause of bronchitis, emphysema and cancer. Even bronchitic patients continue to smoke because the addiction to nicotine is so great. The nicotine has got a hold on them.

To help you to quit smoking, you are advised to enlist the assistance of Stop Smoking clinics; even hypnosis is a viable alternative. The American Cancer Society and the National Cancer Institute provide several types of programs to help you stop smoking. Local cancer societies usually provide a list of programs that can help you stop smoking. Consult your physician for advice on nicotine tablets, patch, gum or nasal spray that can be of value to some individuals. If you are like most smokers, you cannot motivate yourself. Get help now!

TESTS REQUIRED

1. Resting electrocardiogram (ECG or EKG).
2. A stress test.
3. Chest X-ray.
4. Nuclear scans.
5. Echocardiogram.
6. For some patients, coronary arteriography (arteriograms or angiograms) may be required.

For a description of tests, see Tests for Heart Disease.

Drug Treatment

1. Nitrates.
2. Beta-blockers.
3. Calcium blockers (calcium antagonists).

Nitrates

If you suffer from angina, your doctor will advise that you always carry nitroglycerin with you, even if your requirement has been only two pills a year. Nitroglycerin is a nitrate that is used under the tongue in tablet or spray form. Keep the tablets in a dark bottle and not in a pill box, since opening the box lets in light, which will destroy the effectiveness of the drug within a few weeks. Remove the cotton wool from the bottle so you can see and get at the pills easily when in a hurry. Leave the cotton wool in a stock bottle kept in the refrigerator; these tablets will maintain their strength for more than one year. The tablets in the bottle that is opened often should be good for three months.

Nitroglycerin dilates the veins, especially those in the lower half of the body. Blood stays in these enlarged veins and less blood reaches the heart. The heart then has less blood to pump, the muscle works less, thus requiring less oxygen, and, as a result, the pain is relieved.

Nitroglycerin tablets will work best if you keep the lower half of your body much lower than your head, that is, it is better to sit than to lie flat. You may remain propped up in bed. Nitroglycerin causes expansion or dilatation of the blood vessels in the scalp, and this effect may produce a headache. The headache is not due to an increase in blood pressure; in fact, nitroglycerin dilates the arteries slightly and this causes a small fall in blood pressure. Therefore, you must be careful not to take more than two doses of nitroglycerin and not to walk. Unless you are accustomed to the dosage, you may become dizzy or feel faint and fall.

Nitrate tablets that are swallowed are the oldest preparations available in the treatment of angina. These drugs are low in cost and have no serious side effects. They cause frequent headaches, however, and are less effective than beta-blockers.

Nitroglycerin; Glyceryl Trinitrate

Supplied: Sublingual nitroglycerin tablets: 0.15, 0.3 and 0.6 mg. Sublingual glyceryl trinitrate tablets: 300, 500 and 600 micrograms. Also available as a spray: Nitrolingual spray.

Dosage: Patients are usually advised to start with 0.3 mg; the tablet is placed under the tongue with the patient seated. The drug will not be as effective if the patient is lying down, and if the patient is standing, dizziness or faintness may occur. Thereafter, the usual prescribed dose is 0.3 or 0.6 mg of nitroglycerin or 500 to 600 mcg glyceryl trinitrate.

Cutaneous Nitroglycerins (Patches)

Supplied: Comes as paste or ointment, which must not be massaged into the skin. Slow-release cutaneous preparations in the form of adhesive patches are clean and dry and can be used once daily.

The paste or ointment starts to work in 30 to 60 minutes and lasts from four to a maximum of six hours. The long-acting adhesive patches last from 16 to 20 hours and must be removed every 12 hours.

The skin preparations should not be applied to the forearms, hands or lower legs since it takes longer for the drug to reach the general circulation. These preparations are useful during dental work and for minor or major surgery in patients with coronary heart disease.

Dosage: Skin preparations should be used only for two to 14 days. These drugs are not meant to be used for more than a few weeks except if other drug therapy or surgical intervention is not appropriate. They lose their activity if used for more than 12 hours daily. In addition, these preparations must not be stopped suddenly — for example, after using them for a few days, the dose should be tapered and reduced slowly over the next one to two days. In a few patients, when the drugs are stopped suddenly, angina can become worse.

These preparations are applied for 12 hours and taken off for 12 hours.

The various preparations are listed in Appendix A.

Isosorbide Dinitrate (Isordil)

Supplied: Sublingual tablets to be dissolved under the tongue: 5 mg. Tablets for oral use: 10 mg, 20 mg and 30 mg. Prolonged-action tablets: 40 mg. Prolonged-action capsules: 40 mg.
Dosage: A sublingual 5 mg tablet is dissolved under the tongue before an activity known to produce chest discomfort. The 10 mg tablet is swallowed three times daily on an empty stomach, e.g., one hour before meals. If headaches are not too severe, the drug can be increased to 15 mg three times daily for a few days or weeks, then 30 mg three times daily. The prolonged-action 40 mg preparation is taken once or twice daily. Nitrates are more effective taken at 7 a.m., 12 and 5 p.m. The 12-hour gap without nitrates prevents the body from developing tolerance, which destroys the drug's effectiveness.

Advice and Adverse Effects
The sublingual 5 mg tablets take three to five minutes to become effective, somewhat longer than nitroglycerin; therefore, patients are advised to use nitroglycerin during an attack of angina. The drug's effect lasts from 20 to 60 minutes.

Nitrates cause headaches and dizziness. Nitrates should not be used as first choice in the treatment of angina pectoris, especially since beta-blockers have proven to be effective and reliable. In addition, beta-blockers can prevent death or favorably alter the outcome of a heart attack. The use of oral nitrates, therefore, makes sense in patients who cannot take or do not respond to beta-blockers.

Isosorbide Mononitrate

Supplied: The 5-mononitrate of isosorbide dinitrate has become available.
Dosage: 20 mg after meals, 7 a.m. and 2 p.m. daily. Maintenance: 20 to 40 mg twice daily. Imdur can be taken 60 to 120 mg mg once daily at 7 a.m.

Beta-blockers

Beta-blockers are a group of drugs that reduce the action of adrenaline on the heart and arteries. Beta-blockers decrease the heart rate so that the pulse falls from a resting level of about 72 beats per minute to a range of 50 to 60 beats a minute. Second, they reduce blood pressure and third, they cause the heart muscle to contract less forcefully. All three effects cause the heart muscle to require less oxygen, thus preventing angina.

Apart from nitroglycerin under the tongue, beta-blockers are the most beneficial drugs used in the treatment of angina. They have been in use in the United Kingdom since 1964 and in the United States since 1969. The first and most well-known drug in this group is propranolol (Inderal). Several beta-blockers have been approved by the FDA over the years.

Beta-blockers block the effects of the stimulant stress hormones adrenaline and noradrenaline at the so-called beta-receptor sites present on the surface of cells in the heart and in some blood vessels. They therefore prevent the increase in heart rate, the force of heart muscle contraction and the rise in blood pressure normally produced by these stimulants. Commonly used beta-blockers are acebutolol, atenolol, nadolol, metoprolol, propranolol and timolol.

In patients with angina, at least one coronary artery has a block greater than 75 percent. At rest, sufficient blood reaches the heart muscle. However, during moderate activities, the heart rate and blood pressure increase and the heart muscle contracts more forcefully to do the work because more blood containing oxygen is required. The blockage prevents an adequate supply of oxygen from reaching the muscle. This oxygen lack causes the heart muscle to become painful, and the heart rate and blood pressure may further increase during the stress of pain. Basically, beta-blockers cause the heart muscle to require less oxygen to do the same amount of work. The heart rate multiplied by the systolic blood pressure gives an estimation of the amount of work and oxygen required by the heart muscle. Beta-blockers decrease both heart rate and blood pressure, and therefore less oxygen is required. As well, they cause the heart muscle to contract less forcefully so that less oxygen is used. These drugs divert blood from the areas of the heart that have an abundant supply to the deprived area.

Use of Beta-Blockers

If there are *no* contraindications to the use of beta-blockers, the treatment of angina should be sublingual nitroglycerin plus a beta-blocker preferably given once and, at most, twice daily. The beta-blocker is always started at a very low dose and, over a period of days or weeks, increased to an effective dose. A low dose of pro-pranolol, for example, 20 mg three times daily before meals increasing after a week or two to 40 mg three times daily, is advisable. The doctor will check to be sure that the pulse and blood pressure are stable and that there are no side effects from the medications. If necessary, the dose can be increased to 160 mg long-acting (LA) capsule once daily, or 160 mg in the morning and 80 mg at bedtime. A few patients, 1 in 100, are very sensitive to beta-blockers and their pulse rate decreases to less than 48 per minute. It is extremely rare to learn of patients who come to harm because of a slow heart rate. A heart rate of less than 42 may cause dizziness, and the individual may be forced to lie down. The body quickly compensates and the effects of a 40-mg tablet wear off in about four hours. The doctor usually reduces the dose, or in very few cases, the drug is discontinued. In North America there are more than 10 million individuals who are taking beta-blockers or who are candidates for such therapy.

General Cautions That Relate to All Beta-Blockers

1. *Do not suddenly stop taking beta-blockers.* If you have been taking a beta-blocker for several months, your heart rate and oxygen requirement is controlled in just the same way as the reins that control a horse. If beta-blockers are stopped abruptly, it is similar to cutting the reins; the horse may gallop away. Therefore, the heart rate may increase from the accustomed 55 to 65 per minute to 80 to 90 per minute. It is relatively safe to miss one dose of a beta-blocker, or at the most two doses per week. We certainly do not advise you to miss any doses, but there are always unavoidable circumstances. No harm usually results from one missed dose. However, omitting the drug for two to three days consecutively may precipitate angina. Withdrawal should be gradual over weeks and under the guidance of your doctor.

2. Report shortness of breath or wheezing to your doctor as soon as possible.

3. Beta-blockers must not be used in combination with monoamine oxidase (MAO) inhibitors, drugs used only rarely to treat some types of severe depression.

4. Do not take decongestants or cold or cough remedies

containing epinephrine (adrenaline), phenylephrine or pro-pranolamine. These drugs can cause an increase in blood pressure.

5. The combination of beta-blockers and digitalis (digoxin) is safe.

6. Metoprolol and propranolol are broken down in the liver more rapidly in smokers so that blood levels of the drugs are reduced; thus, the drugs may be rendered useless. Atenolol and nadolol are not broken down in the liver and are not affected by smoking. Timolol has been shown to prevent heart attacks or death in smokers as well as nonsmokers.

7. Alcohol: two pints of beer or three ounces of liquor do not cause any interaction or alteration in effectiveness.

Contraindications

Do not take beta-blockers if you have any of the following:

1. Heart failure: Your doctor will obviously know your problem and will not prescribe the drug if you have heart failure and require treatment for angina. However, the good news is that few patients with angina have heart failure. Beta-blockers can precipitate heart failure in patients with very weak heart muscle function. We must point out that the heart muscle is the strongest muscle in the body. It does more work than any other muscle during an individual's lifetime. Many patients who have had two heart attacks are still able to engage in a brisk two-mile walk or climb three flights of stairs, and some can jog one to three miles. The remaining heart muscle is stronger than the quadriceps muscle of the thigh. The heart muscle is strong enough in about 90 out of 100 patients with angina to allow the use of beta-blockers.

2. Bronchial asthma, severe chronic bronchitis, or emphysema: Some patients with mild chronic bronchitis and for whom beta-blockers are deemed necessary to control angina can use atenolol or metoprolol, which has less effect on the lungs. These two drugs are relatively safe at low doses.

3. Allergic rhinitis: Do not commence beta-blockers during a flare-up of allergic rhinitis.

Side Effects

1. The heart and vessels:
- recipitation of heart failure in patients with a very weak heart muscle, as discussed above.
- Severe slowing of the heart rate to less than 42 beats per minute in rare cases if the dose is not carefully adjusted. This is usually quickly spotted by the symptoms of dizziness and ill feeling, and can be quickly rectified. Hence, in practice this is not a problem.
- Extremely cold hands and feet can occur in about 10 percent of patients. The condition improves immediately on discontinuation of the beta-blocker.

2. The lungs:
- Precipitation of wheezing and difficult breathing in individuals who are known to have allergic asthma or severe bronchitis.

3. The nervous or muscular system:
- Dizziness due to excessive slowing of the pulse and reduction in blood pressure.
- Vivid dreams in about 10 percent of patients taking propranolol. These usually clear when given an alternative medication such as atenolol, timolol or nadolol.
- Mild depression. Occurring in less than 10 percent of patients, it is not a major problem in practice. Since atenolol and nadolol do not get into the brain as does propranolol, they cause fewer problems.
- Weakness and muscle fatigue of varying degree, occurring in about 10 percent of patients. A change from propranolol to metoprolol, atenolol or nadolol is advisable. If symptoms persist and no other cause can be found, beta-blockers should be discontinued. In our own large cardiology practice, we have found fewer than 10 such patients since 1965. Certainly beta-blockers may affect individuals who wish to jog more than two miles, but then, patients with angina do not jog.
- Reduction of libido and impotence. Although it occurs in less than 5 percent of patients, it must be monitored by patient and physician. However, beta-blockers, by decreasing the heart rate, blood pressure and heart work, can be useful if pain is precipitated by intercourse.
- Other side effects: In some patients, insomnia, altered

sleep patterns, nervousness, muscle cramps and muscle joint pains can be caused by pindolol.

Atenolol (Tenormin)

Supplied: Tablets: 25 mg (USA), 50 mg, 100 mg.
Dosage: Start 25 mg daily for about three days, then one 50-mg tablet daily at any time of the day. If the condition warrants, the doctor often starts with 50 mg daily. Food does not interfere with the effectiveness of atenolol. One hundred milligrams may be necessary if angina is not controlled and especially if the blood pressure is elevated.

Metoprolol (Lopressor, Betaloc, Toprol XL)

Supplied: Tablets: 50 mg, 100 mg.
Dosage: 50 mg twice daily, before breakfast and at bedtime, increasing if necessary to 100 mg twice daily in the majority of cases, and in a few cases to 200 mg twice daily.

The drug has advantages over propranolol in patients with mild chronic bronchitis; if beta-blockers are deemed necessary to control angina, metoprolol up to 100 mg twice daily is safer than an equivalent dose of propranolol. Toprol XL has the advantage because it is effective when taken once daily.

Nadolol (Corgard)

Supplied: Tablets: 40 mg, 80 mg, 120 mg and 160 mg.
Dosage: 40 to 160 mg only once daily.

As with atenolol, food makes no difference to absorption, and smoking does not alter effectiveness. After a few days or weeks at 40 mg daily, the drug may be increased to 80 mg and in some patients to 160 mg daily.

Propranolol (Inderal)

Supplied: Tablets: 10 mg, 20 mg, 40 mg, 80 mg.
Dosage: 20 mg three times daily *before meals*, increasing slowly, under the supervision of your doctor, to 120 mg daily. After several weeks, a long-acting capsule of 80 mg or 160 mg of propranolol may be preferable. Most patients with angina should receive 160 to

240 mg before adding a calcium antagonist or an oral nitrate. As emphasized, *smoking destroys the effectiveness of propranolol.*

Calcium blockers (antagonists)

Normally, the muscle in the walls of arteries contracts under the influence of the movement of calcium into the cells. Calcium blockers prevent calcium from moving into the cell, thereby causing relaxation and dilatation of the arteries throughout the body. Calcium blockers are not as effective as beta-blockers. The use of calcium blockers in combination with beta-blockers can improve the lifestyle of patients with angina.

How Do Calcium Blockers Work?

Normally, the muscle in the heart and walls of arteries contracts under the influence of a movement of calcium into the cells. Calcium is transported from the exterior to the interior of cells through a system of tubules called slow calcium channels. Calcium reaches the interior of muscle cells and interacts with specialized proteins in the muscle, which then contract. Calcium blockers block the slow calcium channels; this action prevents calcium from going into the cells, thereby causing the muscle of the heart and arteries to relax. These drugs are also known as calcium channel blockers, calcium entry blockers, slow channel blockers or calcium antagonists.

Nifedipine (Procardia XL, Adalat XL Canada)

Supplied: Tablets: 30 mg, 60 mg, and 90 mg.
Dosage: 30 to 60 mg once daily; up to 90 mg daily if necessary.
Nifedipine is of value in the treatment of:

1. Variant angina (coronary artery spasm). All three available calcium antagonists — nifedipine, verapamil and diltiazem — are equally effective in this rare condition.
2. Stable angina pectoris in the following situations:
   • If beta-blockers are contraindicated.
   • If the response to adequate doses of beta-blockers is good but not completely effective; the addition of a calcium blocker is likely to result in further significant improvement.

Actions, Advice and Adverse Effects

Nifedipine strongly blocks the slow calcium channels and causes intense dilatation of arteries. The drug, therefore, dilates the coronary arteries and the arteries of the limbs and elsewhere. This action causes a reduction in the resistance in the arteries, blood pressure and the work of the heart. By causing less work for the heart, along with dilatation of the coronary arteries, the pain of angina is relieved. The drug has no effect on the electrical system of the heart, and it is safe in patients with electrical disturbances.

There are no absolute contraindications to the use of nifedipine. Dizziness occurs in some 3 to 12 percent of patients. If dizziness occurs, the drug is reduced. Dizziness can be made worse when nifedipine is combined with oral nitrates or nitrate preparations placed on the skin or drugs that lower blood pressure. Edema of the legs occurs in about 5 percent of patients, but this does not indicate heart failure. It is due to dilatation of capillaries in the legs. Headaches and a throbbing sensation in the head occur in some 5 to 10 percent of patients, and occasionally the drug has to be discontinued. Patients should be reassured that the throbbing is not due to an increase in blood pressure but to dilation of the arteries in the scalp. The action is similar to a tablet of nitroglycerin put under the tongue. The headaches or throbbing become less severe after a few weeks of treatment, and the majority of patients can tolerate nifedipine in doses of 30 to 60 mg daily. Mild flushing and burning in the scalp and head and occasional indigestion do occur. The drug does not produce or exacerbate stomach ulcers.

Verapamil (Isoptin)

Supplied: Tablets: 120 mg, 180 mg, and 240 mg.
Dosage: 120 to 240 mg once daily.

Indications:

1. Variant angina (coronary artery spasm), which is rare.
2. Chronic stable angina pectoris that does not respond to beta-blockers, in which case verapamil is an effective alternative.
3. Severe palpitations (paroxysmal atrial tachycardia). Verapamil given intravenously in the emergency room is very effective and restores the heart rhythm to normal.

Actions, Advice and Adverse Effects
Verapamil is a moderately potent vasodilator. Verapamil causes a decrease in the contraction of heart muscle. This action can produce heart failure.

Side effects include constipation, which may be distressing, especially in the elderly. In women, secretion of milk from the breasts (galactorrhea) and a minor degree of liver disturbance may rarely occur.

Verapamil is contraindicated in patients with a very slow pulse rate, heart block, sick sinus syndrome, heart failure, an enlarged heart or poor heart muscle function.

Drug Interactions:

- With beta-blockers: The combination may cause marked reduction of the pulse rate to less than 42 per minute. Also, heart failure can be precipitated.
- With digoxin: Verapamil can increase the level of digoxin in the blood, and when both drugs are used, the physician has to recheck levels of digoxin more frequently and may need to lower the dose of both drugs.
- With amiodarone: This is a drug that is used for the treatment of serious forms of extra beats (ventricular tachycardia) and should not be combined with verapamil.
- With tranquilizers: When combined with tranquilizers, Verapamil may have a sedative effect. In this regard, nifedipine does not cause sedation when used along with tranquilizers.
- Verapamil increases the effects of anticoagulants (blood thinners)

Diltiazem (Cardizem)

Supplied: Tablets: 60 mg; capsules CD, 120 mg, 240 mg, and 300 mg.
Dosage: 60 mg tablets three or four times daily. Cardizem CD: 120, 180 or 240 mg once daily.

Indications

Indications are the same as those listed for verapamil except that the drug is not used in the treatment of paroxysmal tachycardia since its effect is very mild.

Actions, Advice and Adverse Effects

Diltiazem has a similar action to verapamil but is not as powerful. The drug causes headaches and dizziness. Disorientation and occasional, reversible elevation of liver enzymes (transaminases) have been seen in some patients. Constipation may be bothersome.

Amlodipine (Norvasc)

Supplied: Tablets: 5, 10 mg.
Dosage: 5 to 10 mg once daily. Indications are the same as outlined under nifedipine.

ANGIOPLASTY/CORONARY BALLOON

This method of treating coronary heart disease is available in most major centers. The first successful coronary angioplasty was performed by Dr. Gruntzig, now deceased, in Zurich in 1977.

The obstructive plaque of atheroma is crushed at one point in one coronary artery (see Fig. 6). Atherosclerosis, however, usually affects several segments of the coronary arteries (see Figs. 1–3).

As the disease advances, every effort must be made to halt its progress. The individual must try to control all risk factors — smoking must be discontinued; blood pressure must be kept within normal limits; stress must be alleviated; cholesterol should be less than 200 mg (5.2 mmol), and LDL cholesterol less than 100 mg (2.5 mmol). Diet plus drug therapy may be necessary to achieve this goal.

Indications

Patients with severe angina who do not achieve sufficient relief with medical therapy are candidates for angioplasty if they have any of the following:

1. One coronary artery nearly completely obstructed (greater than 75 percent) by a discrete, preferably noncalcified plaque of atheroma. Patients with symptoms and obstruction of the left anterior descending artery or right coronary artery before the artery gives off the first branch are the most ideal candidates (see Fig. 2).

2. With increased experience and now steerable catheter systems, doctors are now able to perform the procedure on patients with a broader range of indications. More difficult obstructions are undertaken by experts in some centers. Success is less likely to occur in patients with obstruction in the circumflex artery or at lower points (distal) in the coronary arteries, where there are irregular bends or turns.

3. Patients with acute heart attacks may have the clot dissolved by drugs such as streptokinase or tissue type plasminogen activator and then undergo coronary angioplasty to crush the plaque of atheroma that often lies beneath the clot.

Contraindications

- A coronary artery bypass surgical team is not available.
- A totally blocked artery cannot be cleared because the catheter cannot be positioned (see Fig. 6).
- Disease of the left main coronary artery before it divides into the anterior descending and circumflex branches presents too great a risk.
- The obstruction is in the terminal part of the artery and cannot be reached by the balloon catheter.
- Diabetics do not often obtain beneficial results. Surgery is more effective.

In about 30 percent of individuals with coronary heart disease, the obstruction in the artery is such that coronary angioplasty cannot be done. It is estimated that about 33 percent of patients who have angina and are suitable for coronary artery bypass surgery are candidates for coronary angioplasty.

PROCEDURE

The procedure, percutaneous transluminal coronary angioplasty (PTCA), is so named because the instrument is passed through the skin (percutaneous) and then through the lumen of the artery (transluminal) into the coronary artery, which is molded into

CORONARY ANGIOPLASTY

FIGURE 6

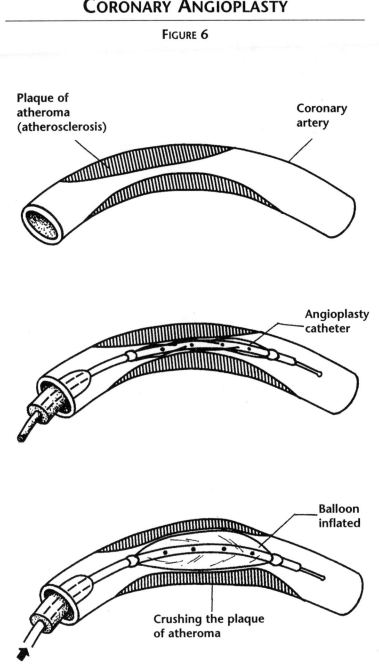

Plaque of atheroma (atherosclerosis)

Coronary artery

Angioplasty catheter

Balloon inflated

Crushing the plaque of atheroma

shape (angioplasty). The balloon-tipped catheter is positioned next to the plaque of atheroma in the artery. The balloon is inflated for 30 to 60 seconds and the plaque is squashed by the pressure (see Fig. 6). The narrowed artery becomes dilated due to splitting (dissection) of the plaque and overstretching of the middle wall (media) of the artery. Transient chest pain may occur during the inflation but is quickly relieved. Several inflations may be necessary to accomplish dilation of the artery. The balloon is then deflated, and dye is injected so that the cardiologist can see if adequate dilation and flow of blood has been achieved.

Following the angioplasty, the patient is monitored in the coronary care unit for 24 to 48 hours. The total hospital stay is usually three days.

OUTCOME OF ANGIOPLASTY

Successful reopening of the artery is achieved in 70 to 90 percent of cases, and with better blood flow, angina improves. The majority of patients return to work seven to 14 days later and have no recurrence of the angina for at least six months. The major early complications include the following: Death occurs in less than 1 percent of cases. A heart attack occurs in approximately 5 percent of cases, because the crushing and splitting of the plaque of atheroma exposes cells and substances that promote blood clotting. Emergency surgery is necessary in about 5 percent of cases, with a 4 to 5 percent mortality. In about 25 percent of patients, it is not possible to pass the catheter through the narrowed area. In about 10 percent, the dilation cannot be accomplished because the plaques are calcified and rock-hard.

These complications are similar to those of coronary artery bypass surgery. The chief late complication at the site of angioplasty is narrowing of the artery (restenosis), in approximately 33 percent of cases. Fortunately, these narrowings can be dilated more easily on the second procedure than on the first. Restenosis occurs in 20 to 35 percent of patients within six months of the procedure, and such patients have a return of their chest pain.

Coronary angioplasty is not in competition with coronary artery bypass surgery. Approximately 50 percent of individuals cannot have coronary angioplasty and must have coronary artery bypass surgery. Coronary angioplasty is much cheaper. The hospital stay is only three days, and patients can usually return to work within one to two weeks. Once the complication of restenosis is over-come, the role of coronary angioplasty will increase.

If you are considering coronary angioplasty, the following sta-tistics will help you and your physician come to a decision: About 40 percent of patients who require coronary bypass surgery are suitable candidates for coronary angioplasty. Some 33 percent of candidates cannot be dilated because the catheters cannot get through to the lesion or cannot crush it because it is rock-hard. Of those who undergo angioplasty, the success rate is 85 percent; they are pain-free and able to do much more work. However, 1 percent die, 3 percent have a heart attack within 24 hours and 3 percent require emergency surgery. Thirty-three percent are blocked (restenosis) within six months and more than half of these can be redilated. Approximately 20 percent usually require coronary artery bypass surgery within the next year.

ANTIHISTAMINES

These well-known antiallergy medications may occasionally cause an increase in the pulse rate because they have an atropine-like effect. In some individuals, the heart rate may become rapid. The sensations called palpitations subside over minutes to hours and usually cause no harm. Patients with angina, however, should be cautious with the use of antihistamines because an increase in heart rate may trigger an attack of angina. Blood pressure is usually not increased by antihistamine use, but many remedies containing antihistamines contain the decongestant phenylpropanolamine, which elevates blood pressure and should be avoided by patients with hypertension and angina.

HISTAMINE ANTAGONISTS

These newer agents differ from the general group of antihista-mines in that they are more selective blockers of specific histamine H1-receptors. They don't produce the bothersome side effects usually noted with antihistamines, such as drowsiness and dry mouth. Unlike antihistamines, they are safe in patients with glaucoma or enlargement of the prostate. Histamine

H1-antagonists include: astemizole and terfenadine. These agents are generally safe, but abnormal heart rhythms, palpitations, transient loss of consciousness and cardiac arrest have been reported.

These agents are broken down in the liver. Thus, patients with liver disease or those using drugs that interfere with liver enzymes, such as the antibiotic erythromycin, may be predisposed to abnormal heart rhythms. Patients taking agents with a similar chemical structure — fluconazole, itraconazole and metronidazole (Flagyl) — may have a greater predisposition to developing bothersome, and even serious, abnormal heart rhythms. Patients with heart disease, those on diuretics or agents that reduce the levels of potassium in the blood, should not take astemizole or terfenadine.

Two newer histamine antagonists, cetirizine and loratadine, have not been noted to cause serious abnormal heart rhythms, but further surveillance and caution is needed in patients with heart disease or in those taking diuretics and other substances that can lower blood potassium. In addition, the antibiotic erythromycin or similar types of antibiotics should not be taken concurrently.

ANTIOXIDANTS

Antioxidants prevent the oxidation of LDL cholesterol, which initiates the atherosclerotic process and its progression to blockage of arteries (see Atherosclerosis/Atheroma). The harmful effect of LDL cholesterol is augmented by oxidized LDL cholesterol particles. Prevention of the oxidation of LDL cholesterol particles by chemical agents is an area of intensive research.

Antioxidant nutrients, particularly vitamin E, vitamin C and beta-carotene, are now widely used with the hope of preventing cancer and heart disease. Although, clinical trials have not shown protection from cancer, the correct "protective" dose may not have been used in some trials. This dose is as yet unknown but is believed to be more than 100 IU daily; 200 to 400 units should suffice. Vitamin E has been shown to increase the immune response; this, in turn, may protect individuals from developing cancer. Benefit is expected only in individuals who take approximately 200 to 400 IU daily for more than two years.

After the past few years of conflicting results, the critical question remains: do antioxidants actually work?

The role of antioxidants in protecting people against heart disease is controversial. The body of evidence is, however, in favor of some beneficial effects, provided that vitamin E supplements of 200 to 400 IU are taken for more than two years. Vitamin C appears to be much less effective than vitamin E in protecting against heart disease. Beta-carotene does not appear to prevent LDL from oxidative modification and has not been shown to have a sufficiently protective role.

Vitamin E is a fat-soluble vitamin found particularly in vegetables and seed oils, particularly soybean, safflower, sunflower seeds, corn, nuts, whole grains and wheat germ. Increased dietary intake has not been shown to decrease the incidence of heart disease or cancer. With aging, however, the vitamin E content of blood platelets decreases; this action may predispose to clumping of platelets and cause a risk of clotting. The elderly may thus benefit from some vitamin supplements.

A large-scale study in the United States showed a reduction in the relative risk of coronary heart disease only in middle-aged women who took vitamin supplements for more than two years. In men, a borderline beneficial effect was observed for those taking above 100 IU daily for over two years. The Health Professionals Follow-Up Study included approximately 40,000 men. This study showed that males who consumed more than 400 IU daily had a 40 percent reduction in the risk of heart disease compared with individuals with the lowest intake of vitamin E. A study involving 121,000 nurses reported a 34 percent decrease in risk of heart disease among women taking greater than 200 IU daily.

Until further clinical trial results are available, 200 to 400 IU daily of vitamin E for more than five years appears to be the best strategy. The beneficial effects of treatments that possess marginal but important beneficial effects may only be observed with correct dosing, and only after several years of intake of the particular substance.

ARTIFICIAL HEART

Despite considerable research and trials in a few courageous patients, such as Dr. Barney Clark in 1982 and Leiff Stenberg, the development of a permanent artificial heart that would be functionally acceptable by patients and physicians is unlikely to be accomplished in the next 25 years. It is imperative that extensive research continues so that this time frame can be shortened. It is surprising that the small human heart, which works so wonderfully in many for more than 80 years, cannot be duplicated despite our advances in technology and space programs.

Patients with terminal, intractable heart failure awaiting heart transplants suffer because of the lack of suitable donors. It is unlikely that in the era of AIDS the source of donors will increase. A production of a functional artificial heart, driven by atomic energy or a suitable small power source that can easily be carried by the patient, is essential. The development of a drive system is a most complex issue. Artificial hearts are driven with compressed air by very large, cumbersome systems outside the body, or by small, portable battery-powered drive systems. The permanent effects of the latter are uncertain. Current research is being directed mainly at systems used as a temporary bridge to heart transplantation. Perhaps by the year 2020, we may have a small enough heart with a sufficiently small power source to implant. A power source that is rechargeable once a year is on the horizon.

ASPIRIN FOR HEART DISEASE

HISTORICAL REVIEW

You do not have to believe in Adam and Eve to recognize the significance of an apple. The old saying *"an apple a day keeps the doctor away"* has been changed to *"an aspirin a day keeps the doctor away"* (see Fig. 7).

Aspirin contains salicylic acid. As early as AD 500, Hippocrates tried to relieve the pain of his patients by asking them to chew willow bark, which contains salicylic acid. In 1763, Reverend Stone of Chipping Norton, in England, showed the benefit of willow bark for individuals with ague-fever. The use of salicylic acid, however, did not materialize until 1853 when Von Gerhardt of Bayer developed Aspirin and in 1899, Felix Hoffman, a Bayer chemist, used Aspirin to treat his father's rheumatism.

The first clinical trial of aspirin in patients dates from 1948-1956: a general practitioner, Lawrence Craven, treated 1,500 relatively healthy, overweight, sedentary men aged 40-65. The result of the study reported in the *Mississippi Valley Journal* concluded that one aspirin a day was sufficient because none of Dr. Craven's 1,500 patients experienced a heart attack over the five-year course of treatment. This small study, however, did not influence physicians to prescribe aspirin to patients for heart problems.

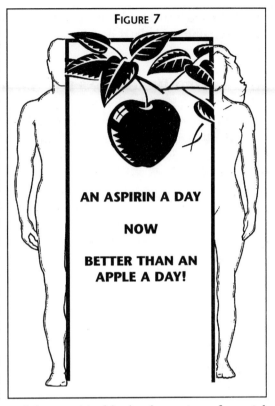

FIGURE 7

AN ASPIRIN A DAY

NOW

BETTER THAN AN APPLE A DAY!

Credit must be given to John Vane working in England in 1971. Dr. Vane showed that aspirin blocks the action of special substances in the body called prostaglandins. This action of aspirin prevents blood platelets from clumping together to produce a clot. Thus, aspirin is referred to as a mild blood-thinner.

The timely 1983 study by Lewis and others in the United States heralded a new era, and aspirin became widely known as a life-saving drug. These physicians showed that one Alka-Seltzer containing 325 mg of acetylsalicylic acid, given to patients with severe angina (heart pains), caused a 49 percent reduction in nonfatal and fatal heart attacks. A Canadian study confirmed this observation. In 1988, the second International Study of Infarct Survival (ISIS-2), a study mounted in the United Kingdom, confirmed a marked increase in survival in a large group of patients given 160 mg of plain aspirin within six hours of the onset of chest pain causing a heart attack. In that study, aspirin greatly improved the life-saving effects of streptokinase, a drug used to dissolve clots soon after the occurrence of a heart attack.

Finally, in 1988, a trial in 22,071 male physicians aged 40 to 80 given 325 mg of aspirin on alternate days for five years demonstrated that aspirin use could result in a 44 percent reduction in fatal and nonfatal heart attacks.

RECOGNIZED INDICATIONS FOR ASPIRIN AND DOSE

- As a life-saving measure when taken within a few hours of chest pain or symptoms resulting from a developing heart attack. Dose: one plain 325 mg tablet of aspirin, chewed and swallowed.
- Unstable angina (severe recurrent chest pains): to prevent heart attack or death. Dose: 325 mg enteric coated aspirin daily.
- Stable angina: mild or recurrent chest pain, usually on exertion: aspirin is used to prevent heart attack or death. Dose: 160 to 325 mg enteric coated aspirin daily.
- After a heart attack to prevent further heart attacks or death. Dose: 160 to 325 mg enteric coated aspirin daily.
- After coronary artery bypass surgery to prevent blockage of the graft. A dose of 325 mg daily is useful for the first few years.
- Men over age 45 or women over age 60 with risk factors: family history of heart attacks before age 60, high cholesterol levels, or LDL cholesterol greater than 160 mg (4 mmol), mild hypertension or diabetes. Dose: 80 mg daily. Bayer produces an 81 mg enteric coated Aspirin that is ideal because a larger dose causes a risk of bleeding from the stomach with long-term use.
- To prevent stroke, see Stroke.

Many individuals worldwide who fall into the above categories are not treated with aspirin by their physicians. It is remarkable that after many years of research, and with the expenditure of several billion dollars, only four of the more than 100 drugs administered by mouth to treat heart diseases cause prolongation of life. These agents are aspirin, beta-blockers, ACE inhibitors and the cholesterol-lowering drugs, statins. "Thus an aspirin a day is now better than an apple a day" (see Fig. 7). Figure 8 indicates that there is no love without a heart. An 81 or 325 mg enteric coated dose of aspirin at bedtime is good protection for those considered at risk.

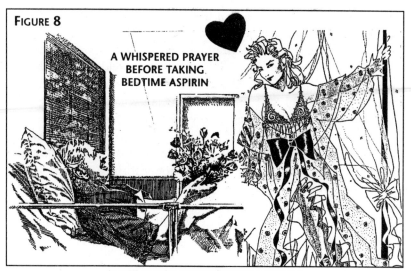

FIGURE 8

A WHISPERED PRAYER
BEFORE TAKING
BEDTIME ASPIRIN

THERE IS NO LOVE WITHOUT A HEART!

ATHEROSCLEROSIS/ ATHEROMA

Atherosclerosis is a form of arteriosclerosis. The latter denotes a hardening of arteries due to all causes, including calcification, loss of elasticity, atheroma and others. The word "atheroma" is derived from the Greek stem "athera," meaning porridge or gruel. When a plaque of atheroma is cut, one can see a gelatinous, thick, porridge-like material that contains cholesterol and other fatty material. The plaque of atheroma involves the inner lining (intima) and the middle wall of the artery (Fig. 3). Apart from a rich fat content, the plaque has a preponderance of smooth muscle cells that are derived from the middle part of the arterial wall (media). These smooth muscle cells are believed to be very important in the formation and growth of the plaque. Substances such as cholesterol and products released from blood platelets stimulate the smooth muscle cells to proliferate, thus enlarging the plaque.

A cross section of a healthy coronary artery is shown in Figure 3. As you can see, the inner wall of the artery in contact with the blood is smooth. When atherosclerosis occurs, a plaque of atheroma juts into the lumen of the artery. The silky smooth lining of the arteries is damaged by the force of blood as it moves through arteries that are elastic and constantly moving in pulsation. With every pulse wave, the arterial wall yields and stretches; over many years some damage must occur. The damage is partially repaired by small blood particles (platelets), which clump together and plug the damaged surface. These platelet plugs form a temporary patch, just like the plug of coagulated blood you see when you nick yourself and a very small clot forms. In the coronary arteries or aorta, small clots are commonly formed on the lining. Presumably, these clots are involved in the repair of injuries to the smooth lining of the arteries. These small blood clots are somehow welded into the lining as hard thickened areas (fibrous plaques). The artery is trying to strengthen its wall in this repair job.

The plaques of atheroma are sometimes smooth, bumpy, large, rough and even ulcerated. Because the vessel wall gets hard (sclerosed), the term used for the disease is atherosclerosis (see Angina Causes). A heart attack is caused by blockage of a coronary artery, and such a blockage is usually due to one or more of the following:

- A blood clot forms on a plaque of atheroma (see Fig. 3). The plaque may be fissured (ulcerated or ruptured), and this often leads to clotting.
- A large plaque of atheroma nearly completely blocks the artery.
- Small blood particles (platelets) may stick to the surface of the plaque in clumps similar to sludge in pipes. The clumped material may dislodge and be wafted downstream by the blood and may block a smaller artery.
- A coronary artery may go into spasm, especially at the site of a plaque, blocking the vessel for a few minutes or a few hours (coronary artery spasm).
- An increase in adrenaline can be produced under the influence of stress or other inciting factors and can cause clumping of platelets that may lead to clot formation. Excess adrenaline from any source can also produce electrical disturbances in the heart, especially ventricular fibrillation. In fibrillation the heart muscle stops contracting and quivers; therefore no blood is pumped, or cardiac arrest.
- The exact mechanism that leads to the formation of blockage by atheroma has defied medical research for the past 60 years. It is certain that a high level of LDL cholesterol, partic-

ularly oxidized LDL (bad) cholesterol, initiates and perpetu-
ates atheroma formation and progression.

- Atherosclerosis causes blockage of arteries and is the cause
of heart pain, angina, heart attacks and death from coronary
heart disease. Blockage of arteries by atherosclerosis is the
basic cause of heart attacks, stroke, aneurysm of the aorta
and poor circulation in the legs.

In the Western world, the UK, Europe, Ireland and Russia,
atherosclerosis is the most common disease affecting men aged 35
to 75 and women 65 to 85. Death due to atherosclerosis is several
times more common than all forms of cancer. The underlying
atherosclerotic disease of the heart's coronary arteries leads to more
deaths than any other disease in industrialized countries. This disease is much more common in young men than women. Women
are fortunately protected from atherosclerosis up to age 55 because
of their ovarian production of estrogens. Because men commonly
die from heart attacks at age 40 to 60, the disease in the left anterior
coronary artery has been appropriately labeled "the widow-maker."

Athlete's Heart

Individuals who partake in regular high levels of exercise for several years develop adaptations in the cardiovascular system. These
features include:

- A slow heart rate of less than 60 beats per minute called sinus
bradycardia. Well-trained athletes often have resting heart
rates of 36 to 44 beats per minute. The heart rate accelerates
to 120 to 140 beats per minute during moderate exercise and
returns to levels less than 60 beats per minute within minutes
of discontinuing exercise. Exercise training causes an increase
in the activity of the vagal nerve that innervates the heart. The
vagus nerves are like the reins of a horse and like good reins,
they operate to slow the heart beat.
- An increase in the bulk, or mass, of the heart muscle occurs,
particularly that of the left ventricle. The small degree of
heart enlargement is a normal physiological response to

regular high levels of exercise over years. The electrocardio-gram in these individuals may indicate the presence of left or right ventricular hypertrophy, or enlargement, and this can be confirmed by echocardiography.

Sudden cardiac death in young athletes is not related to the presence of the very slow heart rates or enlargement of the heart muscle described above. In individuals less than age 35, sudden death is usually caused by unsuspected heart disease, particularly, obstructive cardiomyopathy. In individuals over age 40, coronary heart disease is the usual cause (see Cardiomyopathy or heart muscle disease).

ATRIAL FIBRILLATION

This term is used to describe an abnormal rhythm of the heart-beat. Instead of beating as regularly as a clock, the heart beats very erratically. The very irregular heartbeats may speed up, and the heart rate may be as fast as 150 to 180 beats per minute. These fast and strong beats may be sensed as palpitations. Atrial fibrilla-tion is the commonest persistent heart rhythm abnormality. For a more detailed description of atrial fibrillation, see Palpitations.

BETA-BLOCKERS

The surfaces of cells in various organs and tissues have receptor sites. Hormones and other chemicals react at their respective receptor site to bring about a particular action in the cell. Adrenaline and noradrenaline are called catecholamines and are released from sympathetic nerve endings and as hormones from the adrenal glands. They have their major actions on receptor sites called beta-receptors. Stimulation of the sympathetic-adrenal system during danger or severe stress, for example, causes an outpouring of adrenaline and noradrenaline into the blood circu-lation and at nerve endings. Catecholamines are stimulants and cause an increase in the force of contraction of the heart, and increase heart rate, blood pressure and blood sugar. An outpouring of catecholamines is necessary to prepare the body for a fight-or-flight response. Therefore, we need this surge of adrenaline if we have to flee from a charging bull. While adrenaline and noradrenaline have good effects, in excess they have bad effects and cause overcharging of the cardiovascular system.

It is well documented that during a heart attack large quantities of noradrenaline are released into the heart muscle and can precipitate abnormal heart rhythms, in particular, ventricular fibrillation, during which the heart "quivers," i.e., stops beating, and death occurs. Adrenaline causes an increase in heart rate and an increase in blood pressure and thus causes the heart to work harder. Because a coronary artery is blocked during a heart attack, the increased work with less oxygen available causes further damage to the heart muscle and increases the size of the muscle damage, thus causing a larger heart attack.

By definition, beta-blockers block beta-receptors. Structurally they resemble the catecholamines (adrenaline and noradrenaline) and block the action of these catecholamines at their receptor sites. Thus, heart rate is reduced, resulting in a slower pulse; the force of heart muscle contraction is reduced; blood pressure is lowered, heart rhythm stabilizes and the risk of ventricular fibrillation is significantly reduced. Beta-blockers cause the heart muscle to work less, thus requiring less oxygen, and in time of oxygen lack, such as during a heart attack or severe angina, this action can be life-saving. Because of the reduction in the oxygen requirement of the heart muscle, the beta-blocking drugs are effective in preventing the chest pain of angina pectoris. Since patients with angina have a high risk of developing a heart attack over ensuing years, beta-blockers are important for both pain and prevention. In addition, beta-blockers alter clotting factors and thus may prevent a buildup of sludge, or clotting of blood, without causing bleeding.

An increase in adrenaline such as that produced during stress or vigorous exercise causes an increase in (1) the number and stickiness of blood platelets, (2) a clotting factor (factor VIII, hemophilic factor) and (3) the viscosity of the blood. Beta-blockers block the effect of adrenaline and noradrenaline, and thus may prevent the formation of a blood clot.

Well-run clinical trials have documented that beta-blockers significantly prevent death in patients who are given the drug from the first week of the heart attack and for an additional two years.

In the superbly well-conducted Norwegian study, 1,884 patients were divided at random into two groups. The first group of 942 patients were started on a beta-blocker, timolol, seven days after their heart attack. The other group received a placebo. At the end of two years, the treated group had a 35 percent reduction in heart death, 28 percent reduction in new heart attack, and 65 percent reduction in sudden death. The results are statistically significant. The American Beta Blocker Heart Attack trial gave similar if not just as impressive results.

It is interesting to note the good effect of beta-blockers on the arterial system. The thousands of miles of arteries are constantly under pressure from the pulsatile force and velocity of blood as well as blood pressure. Atherosclerosis is commonly seen where arteries divide. Beta-blockers reduce blood pressure as well as the force and velocity of blood flow at these points of mechanical stress and provide some protection from vessel wall injury. This favorable effect is of paramount importance in patients with high blood pressure. Mechanical injury from the velocity and force of blood is the prime cause of vessel wall injury, which leads to atherosclerosis, dissection of the plaques of atheroma and subsequent thrombosis, as well as rupture of an aneurysm (see Aneurysm).

The name of the game is *preventing heart attacks, as well as preventing death*. Beta-blockers and aspirin are proven by studies in man to prevent death from heart attack. In addition, about 450,000 heart attack patients survive to leave hospitals in the United States and Canada annually, and about 100,000 of these patients will have another heart attack in the following year. Beta-blockers can prevent a heart attack in approximately 30 percent (30,000) of these patients. It is worth your while to get this protection.

For the clinical trials that substantiate the good effects of beta-blockers in post-heart attack patients and the reason why some doctors are reluctant to prescribe them, see Heart Attacks. The beta-blockers that are available and used to prevent fatal or nonfatal heart attacks and in the management of angina or hypertension are given in Appendix A.

The prevention of fatal or nonfatal heart attacks requires a lot of work on the part of doctors and the public. It is your body, and you can work to protect it from the big killers: heart attack, hypertension and stroke. Our discussion should indicate to you that there are no easy answers. Magazine articles and some popular books are often superficial or full of gimmicks and quick fixes that can mislead people.

Prevention requires:

1. *Efficient control of the risk factors* — high blood cholesterol, hypertension, smoking and stress.
2. More attention to the *prevention of blood clotting* to prevent coronary thrombosis. This goal requires:
    - Eating foods that can prevent the formation of clots.
    - The use of drugs that decrease blood clotting without causing bleeding, for example, half to one aspirin daily. Similar and more effective drugs are being tested and will soon become available; so there is hope.
3. *Beta-blocking drugs* for those at moderate to high risk, i.e., patients who have experienced heart attacks, angina or hypertension.

We strongly recommend that you use this information in conjunction with the advice of your doctor to gain maximum protection and thus prevent a heart attack.

BLOOD CLOTS

The cause of a fatal or a nonfatal heart attack in 90 percent of cases is a blood clot in a coronary artery (coronary thrombosis). The clot often occurs on the surface of a plaque of atheroma that is partially obstructing the lumen of the coronary artery. Patients may have many large atheromatous plaques and yet not develop a clot over a five- to 15-year period. There is no test that can tell us when and where a clot will occur. This is the $64,000 question. If we can fly to the moon, you would think that such a question could be answered.

Cholesterol, hypertension and cigarette smoking have little to do with the clotting of blood; therefore, we must look elsewhere. We are convinced that unless we do something to help the population at risk to prevent a blood clot from forming in the coronary arteries, we will not have a major reduction in fatal and nonfatal heart attacks.

Recently, cardiologists have started to use drugs to dissolve clots in the coronary arteries. In many centers in North America, when a patient is admitted with a heart attack within three hours of onset of chest pain, the doctor will inject the thrombolytic drugs streptokinase, tPA, or reteplase, which have been shown to dissolve freshly formed clots. When a clot prevents blood from reaching part of the heart muscle, this area of the heart muscle dies within a half to one hour. Therefore, you should get to the hospital as quickly as possible if you suspect you are having a heart attack. After six hours, dissolving the clot may not help because it is too late. Therefore, we should try to prevent the clot from forming.

Small particles, platelets, are present in the blood and circulate as elliptical flat disks. Platelets are the first defense of the body against excessive bleeding. At the site of bleeding, platelets accumulate and stick together to form a clump to plug the seepage of blood. When the platelets clump together, other clotting factors come into play with the final conversion of a blood protein, fibrinogen, which turns into a mesh of fibrin strands that traps red cells and additional platelets, thus forming a firm clot.

CAUSES

Blood clots are believed to occur in the coronary artery because of the following:

- Platelets become sticky when they come in contact with the damaged lining of blood vessels. Platelets interact with the damaged surfaces, and chemicals that are produced at the site cause the platelets to clump and form a clot. Chemicals in the body that cause platelets to clump or sludge include collagen from the damaged vessel wall, adrenaline and a very powerful platelet-clumping chemical called thromboxane A2. Platelets are most sticky when they are newly released from the bone marrow. This may occur four to 14 days after any type of surgery. For example, there is a higher incidence of clots in veins of the legs after surgical operations. The lack of movement of the legs causes a slowing of the circulation in veins and increases the chances of a clot in the deep veins of the legs.
- Mild cooling and chilling of the body without hypothermia can lead to an increase in the total number and stickiness of

platelets and may increase clotting. This may influence the incidence of coronary thrombosis in winter.

- During stress, adrenaline and other chemicals produced increase the number and stickiness of platelets, which may clump on to atheromatous plaques.
- Certain foods, especially high-fat foods, increase the stickiness of platelets and influence other blood-clotting factors, but to a small extent.
- Atheromatous plaques produce turbulence and slow the blood flow in the coronary artery. The force of blood and increases in blood pressure can cause fissures or rupture of plaques. Platelets stick to these areas on the plaque and can start clot formation.
- Prevention of clots will be achieved if we prevent formation of atheromatous plaques and their rupture. Rupture of a plaque liberates substances that rapidly cause clotting and blockage of arteries.
- Nicotine and carbon monoxide, which are by-products of cigarette smoking, increase platelet stickiness and may be important factors.
- Some foods have a high vitamin K content and increase the concentration of a clotting factor made in the liver (prothrombin). In addition, fibrinogen, the final protein involved in the formation of clots, is manufactured in the liver, and it has been shown that the mean fibrinogen concentration and viscosity in the blood is increased in patients who have had heart attacks. Thus we believe that certain foods other than those involved in elevating blood cholesterol may be important in increasing or decreasing clot formation (see Linolenic Acid under Cholesterol).

NONDRUG TREATMENT

We strongly recommend the following dietary measures:

a. Eat less fatty meals, thereby reducing your saturated fat and hydrogenated fat intake. Saturated fats form LDL (bad) cholesterol in the body.
b. Try to increase the intake of foods that may prevent blood clotting; in particular, onions, garlic and foods containing alpha-linolenic and eicosapentaenoic acids; the latter derived

from fish and cod liver oil. The latter polyunsaturated acid in the diet of fish-eating Japanese and Inuit prevents clumping of platelets and has favorable effects on the blood-clotting system. These foods decrease platelet clumping as well as increase vessel wall prostacyclin (prostaglandin), a compound that helps to keep the lining of the artery clean. Increase your consumption of fish, for example, mackerel and salmon, which have a high content of the polyunsaturated fatty acids. Linolenic acid is of proven value in prevention (see Linolenic Acid under Cholesterol).

c. Avoid or use sparingly: alfalfa, turnip greens and broccoli, which are very high in vitamin K, and lettuce, cabbage and spinach, which have a moderate content. The concentration of prothrombin, a bloodclotting factor, can be increased by foods containing high amounts of vitamin K. If you are taking the blood thinners warfarin or Coumadin, use these foods in moderation and not erratically. Your doctor will find it more difficult to thin your blood and more frequent blood tests may be necessary.

- See Heart Attack Prevention Diet.

DRUG TREATMENT/BLOOD THINNERS

- Aspirin
- Dipyridamole
- Ticlopidine
- Anticoagulants

The first three drugs prevent platelet clumping (aggregation). They are not blood thinners (anticoagulants) and do not cause spontaneous bleeding.

Aspirin

Supplied: Aspirin blocks an enzyme (cyclo-oxygenase) within the blood platelets and prevents the formation of thromboxane A2, which causes clumping of platelets. A dose of aspirin as low as 80 mg daily, a quarter of an ordinary aspirin, is capable of blocking the formation of thromboxane A2. A dose of 325 mg (one ordinary aspirin) stops platelet clumping for two to five days. Clinical trials have confirmed that a small dose of aspirin, 160 to 325 mg daily soon after a heart attack, can prevent heart attacks and death.

Dosage: We advise patients with coronary heart disease or those at risk to take a 325 mg coated or 81 mg of aspirin daily (see the general section on Aspirin).

Dipyridamole

Supplied: Tablets: 50 mg, 75 mg.
Dosage: 50 to 75 mg three times daily one hour before meals.

This drug is not useful when used alone, but in combination with aspirin, has been shown to reduce the incidence of clotting of coronary artery bypass grafts (CABG). In animal experiments, the drug has been shown to be effective in preventing platelet clumping. Rats stressed with electric shocks developed platelet clumping in the coronary arteries, which produced small areas of damage to the heart muscle (myocardial infarcts). This damage can be prevented in more than 80 percent of animals when pretreated with dipyridamole. Aspirin and sulfinpyrazone have similar effects.

During the 1970s a clinical trial called the Paris-1 Study evaluated the usefulness of dipyridamole combined with aspirin in about 2,000 patients who had had heart attacks. This study cost about $20 million to complete and unfortunately included patients with old and very old heart attacks, that is, ranging from six months to three years. Only patients with less than a six-month-old heart attack showed a significant reduction in death rate, but this is not acceptable scientific evidence.

The combination of dipyridamole and aspirin was re-evaluated in a 1980 to 1984 clinical trial. Three thousand patients were treated within 30 days of their heart attacks and followed for two years.

The combination was not of value in preventing deaths due to heart attacks, but caused a 37 percent reduction in the recurrence of heart attacks. The combination of aspirin and dipyridamole prevents formation of blood clots in vein grafts of patients who have had a coronary artery bypass graft. Some surgeons may advise you to take the combination of aspirin and dipyridamole for several years. Recent trials have shown that 326 mg of aspirin is as good as the combination. Dipyridamole is not effective when used without aspirin.

Ticlopidine

Ticlopidine inhibits platelet clumping and can decrease the frequency of chest pain as well as correct abnormal ECG changes in patients with attacks of angina due to coronary heart disease. Studies implicate platelets as a major culprit in the causation of complications of coronary heart disease, including fatal or nonfatal heart attacks or angina. This drug is used in patients to prevent stroke if aspirin is not tolerated, but can damage white blood cells.

Anticoagulants (Warfarin, Coumadin)

Anticoagulants (blood thinners) are not significantly effective in preventing a first or recurrent heart attack. They were used for this purpose from 1955 and abandoned from 1968. They are used successfully for the treatment of clots in:

- Leg veins
- The lungs (pulmonary embolism)
- The heart chambers (atrium or ventricle), especially if such clots move from the heart and block an artery elsewhere in the body such as in the legs or brain. Fortunately, the latter occurrence is rare. Warfarin is commonly used for the prevention of stroke in patients with atrial fibrillation.

BLOOD PRESSURE

The heart pumps blood directly into blood vessels called arteries, which are like a series of pipes. The narrower the arteries, the greater the resistance or impedance to the flow of blood; therefore the heart must pump with greater force. The amount of force with which the blood is being pumped from the heart through the arteries is the blood pressure. The blood exerts pressure against the artery walls, thus the term "blood pressure." Everyone has blood pressure, and we will discuss later what is meant by high blood pressure.

The pressure in the arteries when the heart contracts (systole) is called systolic blood pressure. Usually this is less than 140 millimeters (mm) Hg (mercury). The pressure in the arteries when the heart is relaxed (diastole) is called diastolic pressure, and this is usually less than 90 mm Hg. Another way of looking at blood pressure is as follows: Each contraction of the heart causes blood to be pushed (propelled) through the arteries in the form of a pulse wave; thus the flow of blood in the arteries is pulsatile. A wave must have a crest and a trough. The crest is caused when the heart contracts (systole) and is the highest pressure, or systolic blood pressure. The trough is caused when the heart relaxes (diastole), producing the lowest pressure, or diastolic pressure.

The resistance in the arteries against which the heart must pump is called the total vascular resistance. If the total vascular resistance increases, blood pressure increases. This resistance is increased when the arteries are constricted by disease, aging, drugs or naturally occurring chemicals in the body such as adrenaline. The amount of blood expelled by the heart into the arteries in one minute is called the cardiac output and is about five liters per minute. Blood pressure is equal to the total vascular resistance multiplied by the cardiac output. Hypertension is the medical term for high blood pressure and has nothing to do with being hyper, or excessive nervous tension. See Hypertension.

Bundle Branch Block

Right Bundle Branch Block (RBBB)

The electrical bundles that take the electrical impulses to the right ventricle are damaged or do not conduct the impulse; the electrical impulses fail to reach the right ventricle. The diagnosis is made only from the ECG. (See Fig. 16, Electrical System of the Heart, in the section on Palpitations.) The condition is not uncommon and can be seen in normal individuals. The condition does not affect lifestyle and causes no symptoms; it does not lead to heart attacks and requires no treatment. RBBB is most often seen with coronary heart disease, valvular heart disease and lung disease. The heart rate remains normal. A pacemaker is never required.

LEFT BUNDLE BRANCH BLOCK (LBBB)

This condition is not uncommon and is due to a block of the conduction in the bundle that receives impulses from the atrium across the left ventricle (see Fig. 16). The ECG is typical, and the doctor makes the diagnosis only after looking at the ECG. Right bundle branch block is often seen in normal individuals. Left bundle branch block, on the other hand, is more often due to subtle diseases of the heart, including coronary heart disease, valvular heart disease and muscle scars. Left bundle branch block does not cause any disturbance in the heart rate and does not require an artificial pacemaker.

CARDIOMYOPATHY

This is a rare form of heart disease that affects only the heart muscle. The term cardiomyopathy is derived from cardio, the heart, and myopathy indicates a weakness or disturbance of the muscle. Heart muscle diseases of unknown cause are classified under the term cardiomyopathy.

In one form of heart muscle disease, the muscle of the ventricle becomes considerably thickened to the point that the cavity of the left ventricle becomes nearly filled with muscle mass; thus less blood enters the chamber and less blood is expelled into the circulation. Because the muscle is enlarged, or hypertrophied, the disease is called hypertrophic cardiomyopathy. This is a disease of young adults. The muscle enlargement may be so severe that it obstructs the flow of blood into the aorta, and death may occur suddenly, particularly in individuals from age 12 to 36 years. Some athletes who have died suddenly have had this disease. In some families, hypertrophic cardiomyopathy is caused by mutation in the cardiac myosin gene. Approximately 60 percent of cases occur in families with an autosomal-dominant pattern and 40 percent of cases are sporadic.

In another form of heart muscle disease, the heart dilates without increasing the size of the muscle. The chambers are swollen, and the muscle becomes weak. This condition often results in failure of the heart to pump blood, which results in heart failure. Heart transplants are required in some of these patients. See Heart Failure.

Other types of heart muscle diseases may be caused by viruses. Recently, patients with AIDS have had HIV viral infection of the heart muscle. The heart muscle may be damaged by cocaine, an overload of iron (hemochromatosis) and some inherited conditions.

CARDIOPULMONARY RESUSCITATION (CPR)

Perhaps you may happen to be near someone who falls to the ground and stops breathing. You may be alone or someone summons you to help. Can you help? If you have never learned how to do CPR, you will not know what to do to save a life. Thus it is wise for all individuals to attend a practical course in CPR or at least read and practice the drill until it becomes automatic. The technique is really quite simple. Your main goal in applying CPR is trying to get oxygen to the individual's brain to keep it alive until expert help arrives. We have summarized the points to assist you when faced with an individual who has "dropped dead" in your presence so that you may render some valuable assistance.

Patients may lose consciousness and fall because of several reasons:

- A simple faint. The patient has a pulse, does not stop breathing and has no shaking of the limbs. Simply keeping the head down, preferably with the individual lying flat, and raising the legs up in the air above the patient's hips will cause blood to flow from the legs. In 30 seconds to one minute, the individual will recover completely.
- A seizure (epilepsy). The patient's limbs show typical movements that are jerky, the limbs get rigid, and there is a combination of rigidity and jerking of one or more limbs. The patient is breathing, but saliva and foam bubble from the mouth; some individuals pass urine or stools; recovery is the norm.
- A stroke. During a stroke, circulation to part of the brain is cut off because of a blood clot in an artery in the brain. Strokes usually occur in individuals over age 60. It is rare for the patient to fall suddenly to the floor without some

warning. The patient will have a pulse, and breathing will be present. Unlike with a simple faint, elevating the limbs, which should be tried, is not successful over a period of one to two minutes. There is no reason to do CPR since the heartbeat, circulation and respirations still exist.

- Cardiac arrest. During cardiac arrest, the heart stops beating completely and is at a standstill (asystole) in about 25 percent of individuals. In about 75 percent, the cardiac arrest is due to ventricular fibrillation, during which the heart muscle does not contract, but quivers. During ventricular fibrillation, there is no effective heart contraction, and blood is not pumped to the brain or other parts of the body. Ventricular fibrillation can be treated by an electrical shock, which defibrillates the heart and replaces the ventricular fibrillation with a normal heartbeat. In standstill or asystole, there is no electrical current in the heart, and using electrical shock is of no value. In a few cases, the heart may commence beating on its own; the condition is called a Stokes-Adams attack, named after the doctors who first described it. A few can be saved by the insertion of a pacemaker if the attack is in the hospital.

It is wise for a family member of a heart patient to know how to give CPR. It reassures the patient that possibly something can be done. The knowledgeable individual also feels some sense of confidence, which promotes hope.

CPR is only a temporary measure. The aim is to get blood containing a fresh supply of oxygen to the brain. Therefore, you need to breathe enough air into the patient's lung, then compress the chest to cause the nonbeating heart to expel blood into the arteries, thus producing circulation of the blood to the brain. The rare patient may be revived, and the heart begins to beat spontaneously. In those with ventricular fibrillation, death will occur unless the heart is defibrillated. Therefore, the $64,000 question is, Does the ambulance have a portable defibrillator and a team that can defibrillate the patient? If so then there is hope.

The principles and methods of CPR are simple to apply. You should also contact your local heart association or the Red Cross to find out where CPR courses are held.

How to Recognize Cardiac Arrest

Determine:

- That the patient is *unconscious* and is unresponsive to shaking or commands.
- The patient is *not breathing.* You should verify this.
- There is *no pulse.* Check for a pulse by feeling the carotid artery in the neck. The right carotid artery is felt one inch from the angle of the jaw. Place your index finger in a straight line next to (parallel with) the windpipe (trachea) so that the entire length of the first finger pad is touching the skin. The tip of the index finger should be approximately opposite the Adam's apple. You can start by feeling the most prominent part of the Adam's apple with the tips of two fingers, then slide the finger outward to reach the grove between the hard cartilage of the windpipe and the muscle of the neck. The carotid artery lies only a few millimeters under the skin, and the pulsation is easily felt. Practice feeling this pulse so that you can find it in a hurry, taking no more than 10 seconds. Therefore, within 30 seconds you should have arrived at a conclusion that a cardiac arrest has occurred. Speed of diagnosis is critical. Within three to four minutes of cardiac arrest, irreversible brain damage can occur because of lack of oxygen. The resuscitation procedures listed below follow the recent recommendations of the American Heart Association.

Your intention is to provide basic life support until advanced life support in the form of expert technical help arrives. Basic life support consists of the recognition of cardiac arrest and the proper application of cardiopulmonary resuscitation to maintain life until advanced life support is available.

The A-B-C Steps of CPR

The A-B-C steps of CPR should be commenced immediately. Quickly turn the victim flat on the back on a hard surface (preferably the floor).

A: AIRWAY. Use the head-tilt/chin-lift maneuver to open the airway and determine that the victim is not breathing. Place one

THE ABC OF CARDIOPULMONARY RESUSCITATION

FIGURE 9

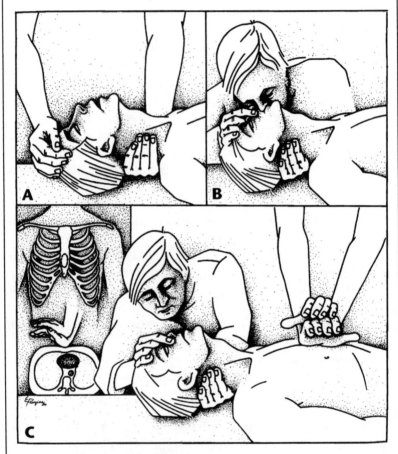

A The airway is opened.
B Breathing: The victim's nostrils are pinched closed
   and the rescuer breathes into the victim's mouth.
C Circulation: If no pulse is present, external chest
   compression is instituted.

hand on the victim's forehead and apply firm, backward pressure with the palm to tilt the head back (see Fig. 9). Put your index and middle fingers of the other hand under the bony part of the lower jaw. Lift the chin forward and support the jaw, thus helping to tilt the head back. Do not use your thumb for lifting the chin and do not press your fingers into the soft tissue under the chin.

The head-tilt/chin-lift maneuver should bring the teeth almost together and maintain dentures in position. Now place your ear over the victim's mouth and nose. If you do not hear or feel the flow of air escaping and the chest does not rise and fall, the victim is not breathing.

B: BREATHING. Pinch the victim's nostrils closed, using your thumb and index finger of the hand on the forehead. Then take a deep breath, make a tight seal over the victim's mouth with your mouth, and blow into the victim's mouth. Blow air into the victim's mouth to fill the lungs (ventilate) rapidly two times. At this point, check for the carotid pulse using the hand that was lifting the chin.

C: CIRCULATION. If there is no pulse, begin compressing the chest. Place the heel of one hand over the lower half (see Fig. 9) of the breastbone but at least one inch (two centimeters or two finger-breadths) away from the end of the breastbone (xiphoid process). Position the heel of your other hand on the top of the first. *Keep the fingers off the rib cage* (see Fig. 9). If your hands are too high, ineffective chest compression may result, and fracture of the ribs may occur. Keep your arms straight at the elbow (locked elbows) and apply pressure as vertically as possible. Your shoulders should be directly above the victim's breastbone. Chest compressions are thus easily carried out by forceful movements of the shoulders and back, so the maneuver is less tiring. Depress the breastbone one to two inches (three to five centimeters) toward the spine, and alternately compress and relax.

You should also apply mouth-to-mouth ventilation in the following way: If there is only a *single* rescuer, use 15 compressions to two ventilations. If there are *two* rescuers, use five compressions to one ventilation. Compress the chest at a rate of 80 to 100 per minute if possible.

CPR should never be interrupted for more than five seconds. It should be continued until skilled help arrives.

Note that the victim's mouth should be almost completely closed. However, depress the lower lip a bit so that the mouth remains slightly opened. If dentures cannot be managed in place, remove them after first giving the very important first two breaths.

You must see the chest rise and fall. There is no logical reason to first look for foreign bodies or vomitus before giving the first two breaths. If the first two breaths meet with resistance and the chest fails to rise when you breathe air into the patient's mouth, make sure that the airway is properly opened by the head-tilt/chin-lift method and that the seal around the mouth is airtight, then clear the airway with your fingers if necessary. The fact that the patient suddenly dropped to the ground and was not choking while eating is sufficient to persuade you not to waste time searching for meat or vomitus.

THE HEIMLICH MANEUVER

This maneuver is used for removing foreign bodies from the airway. You must stand behind and wrap your arms around the waist of a conscious victim. Then place the thumb side of your fisted hand above the victim's navel and well below the lower tip of the breastbone. Using the other hand, forcefully push the fist with a quick upward thrust into the victim's abdomen. Repeat the thrust a few times, if necessary.

An unconscious victim is placed face upwards. The rescuer kneels and places the heel of one hand above the navel and with the second hand on top pushes into the abdomen with a quick upward thrust.

CONCLUSION

You can do your part and learn CPR and encourage groups in your community to do the same. In cities where a rapid-response, 911 emergency care system is used in conjunction with citizens trained in CPR, countless lives have been saved.

The Belfast, Brighton and Seattle services are well known, and their noble example has been followed by cities such as Cleveland, Dallas, Dayton, Houston, Jacksonville, Miami, St. Paul and Washington, D.C. Might not a telethon help this noble cause in other cities?

CHELATION THERAPY

Chelation therapy using EDTA to clear obstructions in the femoral arteries caused by atheroma has not been successful. This therapy has been tried in small numbers of patients from time to time during the past 20 years in nonrandomized trials. A study by van Rij et al reported in the September 1994 issue of *Circulation* states that "chelation therapy has no significant beneficial effects over placebo."

There are no placebo-controlled randomized trials of chelation in patients with coronary heart disease. Patients are warned that they place their lives at risk if they discontinue their proven heart medications for a trial of chelation therapy.

Agents such as EDTA can remove iron from the body but cannot dissolve the plaques of atheroma that obstruct coronary arteries.

CHOLESTEROL

Cholesterol is a lipid, or fat-like substance, made by animal cells. The role of an elevated blood cholesterol in causing a blockage to arteries by atherosclerosis and a subsequent heart attack has been a controversial issue for more than 40 years. Therefore, advice to patients has often been halfhearted. Until recently we were not able to put the blame firmly on cholesterol and convince our colleagues and patients. We were missing the key piece of scientific evidence proving that lowering of elevated blood cholesterol in humans prevents fatal or nonfatal heart attacks.

In 1984, the Lipid Research Clinics Program reported the results of a successful trial in the United States over a period of 10 years at a cost of $150 million. The trial showed that a reduction in blood cholesterol resulted in a small but significant reduction in fatal and nonfatal heart attacks.

The study was randomized, and scrupulously conducted in many centers in the United States and in two centers in Canada. More than 480,000 men aged 35 to 59 were screened to find subjects who had a cholesterol level greater than 265 milligrams (6.9 mmol; see Appendix B for conversion of mg to mmol) but were otherwise healthy and, in particular, had no evidence of heart disease or hypertension. The 3,806 men found suitable for the trial were asked to follow a cholesterol-lowering diet. A random group of half the men were given a drug to lower cholesterol (cholestyramine, 24 g daily); the other half were given an identical-looking but nonmedicinal preparation (placebo). The drug caused an 8 percent lowering of the blood cholesterol. After follow-up for an average of 7.4 years, there were 187 fatal or nonfatal heart attacks in the control group and 155 in the drug-treated group. Unfortunately, cholestyramine is a powder that is mixed with fruit juice and is unpleasant to taste. Patients do not comply with taking it two or three times daily, and it is not surprising that the reduction in cholesterol was 8 percent rather than an expected 25 percent. Nevertheless, the study shows that lowering of cholesterol by a special drug reduces the occurrence of heart attack. Thus a reduction of blood cholesterol by diet should have a similar good effect.

A low-saturated fat diet that will lower blood cholesterol by 10 percent is feasible. Whereas strict dieting can decrease total cholesterol 5 to 10 percent, the newer drugs, **statins, (HMG-CoA reductase inhibitors),** have been documented in clinical trials to decrease total cholesterol and LDL (bad) cholesterol from 15 to 30 percent.

In 1994-1995, randomized clinical trials in sufficient numbers of patients have documented the beneficial results of lowering LDL cholesterol with statins. These studies confirm that a decrease in LDL cholesterol to less than 120 mg (3 mmol) prevents heart attack, deaths and blockage in coronary arteries.

Statins include:

- Fluvastatin (Lescol)
- Lovastatin (Mevacor)
- Pravastatin (Pravachol)
- Simvastatin (Zocor)

What is a normal blood cholesterol, and when does the level produce a risk of coronary heart disease?

Blood cholesterol is not necessarily very high, i.e., greater than 265 milligrams (6.9 mmol), in those who have heart attacks. In fact, most heart attacks occur in individuals with blood cholesterol around the average 220 (5.7 mmol) to 250 mg (6.5 mmol). In the lipid study described above, only 3,806 men with a blood cholesterol greater than 265 mg could be found from a screen of 480,000. The remainder had cholesterol levels of less than 265 mg and likely 200 to 250 mg.

Between 1970 and 1989, laboratories in North America reported a normal cholesterol as being between 150 (3.9 mmol) and 250 (6.5 mmol). But it is now established that individuals with so-called normal cholesterol in the range of 220 to 250 are at increased risk, and heart attacks are common in individuals with such levels. A blood cholesterol of 220 (5.7 mmol) to 250 mg (6.5

mmol) is considered high by world standards and can no longer be considered normal. Most doctors now talk about an optimal level, i.e., a level that can be considered safe. We agree with experts that a total cholesterol level of less than 200 mg (5.2 mmol) or LDL less than 120 mg (3 mmol) is optimal, and heart attacks are uncommon in individuals with a cholesterol level less than 180 mg (4.7 mmol).

If we just treat patients with a cholesterol level greater than 250 mg (6.5 mmol) with nondrug therapy, we will be excluding more than 80 percent of the population who are at high risk. To re-emphasize, most heart attacks in North America occur in people with blood cholesterol between 220 and 260 mg. If your cholesterol is less than 180 mg (4.7 mmol), you obviously deal with cholesterol by your own natural process. You are among the fortunate; no dietary modification is necessary, and your cholesterol need not be rechecked for five years.

Studies that support and finally prove that lowering cholesterol decreases the risk of heart attack and death include:

- The Seven Countries Study included more than 12,000 men from Finland, Greece, Italy, the Netherlands, Japan, the United States and Yugoslavia. The Finns had the highest intake of saturated fat, the highest blood cholesterol levels (greater than 280 mg) and the highest number of fatal and nonfatal heart attacks, about 900 per 100,000. The Japanese, with an average blood cholesterol of 140 mg, had the lowest heart-attack death rate of 102 per 100,000. The United States, with an average of 220 mg, had a heart-attack death rate of 670 per 100,000. The death rate was also low in Greece and Italy. Japanese immigrants to the United States who adopt an American diet have an incidence of coronary heart disease ten times that of their countrymen in Japan.
- The Framingham Study has contributed good evidence to support the view that a high blood cholesterol greatly increases the risk of developing coronary heart disease.
- People who have a rare inherited defect that prevents the body from getting rid of cholesterol may have blood cholesterol levels as high as 1,000 mg from early childhood. These patients develop cholesterol-containing lumps and bumps, especially on the knees, elbows, and tendons of the wrists and the Achilles tendon. These people may have a heart

attack before age 35. Fortunately the condition is rare.

There are several recent studies that confirm that decreasing total cholesterol to below 200 mg (5 mmol) or LDL cholesterol to below 120 mg (3 mmol) decreases the risk of heart attack and death, and reduces the obstruction in arteries. These studies include:

- The Scandinavian Simvastatin Study reported in *Lancet* in November 1994 shows that long-term treatment with simvastatin improves survival in patients with coronary heart disease. In that study, 4,444 patients with angina or previous heart attack, and cholesterol levels ranging from 5.5 to 8 mmol (215 to 312 mg), were randomly selected to follow either a cholesterol-lowering diet or simvastatin, 10 to 40 mg daily, and followed for 5.5 years. There were 189 heart-attack deaths in the dietary (control) group, and 111 in the simvastatin-treated group. Decrease in survival was observed in both men and women. Treated patients benefited from a 37 percent reduction in the risk of undergoing bypass surgery or angioplasty.

- The Multicenter Anti-Atheroma Study of 381 patients with coronary artery disease treated with 20 mg of simvastatin for four years, showed a decrease in new obstructions in coronary arteries, and fewer treated patients required angioplasty or surgery.

- The result of the Pravastatin Limitation of Atherosclerosis in the Coronary Arteries (PLAC1) trial was reported at the American College of Cardiology in March 1994. In that study, 408 patients who had coronary angiograms that showed an obstruction greater than 50 percent were randomly selected to receive either pravastatin or a placebo. At the end of three years, repeat coronary angiograms showed 33 new obstructions in the placebo group, but only 15 new obstructions in the treated patients. Placebo patients' cholesterol levels were approximately 6 mmol (240 mg), and their LDL was 4.2 mmol (165 mg); these levels were significantly reduced by pravastatin treatment.

- The Pravastatin Multinational Study for cardiac risk patients involved more than 1,000 patients. After six months, there were 13 heart attacks in the control group versus one in the treated group.

- A Heart, Lung and Blood Institute Study showed that a reduction in blood cholesterol by the drug cholestyramine tends to prevent enlargement of atherosclerotic plaques in humans. The statins are more effective than cholestyramine.

- The result of the Scotland Coronary Prevention Study was reported in the *New England Journal of Medicine*, November 1995. Pravastatin administered to men 45 to 64 years of age with moderately elevated cholesterol (average 272 mg, 7 mmol), reduced the incidence of heart attack and death from cardiovascular causes. The study randomized 6,595 men and followed them for 4.9 years; 248 nonfatal and fatal heart attacks occurred in the placebo group and 174 in the pravastatin group.

TYPES OF CHOLESTEROL

Cholesterol is an essential part of the fatty sheath that insulates nerves and the outer membrane of cells, and is a component of chemicals that include steroids (cortisone) and sex hormones such as androgens and estrogens.

Some of the cholesterol in blood is derived from the food you eat, but the major part, greater than 70 percent, is manufactured in the liver, mainly from saturated fats. Thus, if we had no cholesterol in the diet, the liver would manufacture more cholesterol to compensate. Some excess cholesterol is excreted in the bile. Cholesterol is present only in foods of animal origin, in particular, eggs, milk, butter, cheese and meats, and a very high concentration is present in gland meats, such as liver, brain, kidney, heart and sweetbread. Plant-based foods such as vegetables, fruits, grains and beans contain no cholesterol.

In order to understand the changes that may be required in your diet, it is important to learn the difference between the types of cholesterol: total cholesterol, low-density lipoprotein (LDL) cholesterol and high-density lipoprotein (HDL) cholesterol. You should also become familiar with the different types of fats in foods: triglycerides, saturated fats, monounsaturated fats and polyunsaturated fats (see Cholesterol and Fats).

Total Cholesterol

Cholesterol is a fat (lipid) that is insoluble in water. Cholesterol absorbed by the intestine or released from the liver into the blood stream does not circulate freely in solution but is attached to a protein carrier, forming a molecule called a lipoprotein. Lipoproteins vary in size and density; the smaller the size, the higher the density. Cholesterol may be transported in a low-density lipoprotein; thus the term "low-density lipoprotein (LDL) cholesterol." There is also a high-density lipoprotein (HDL) cholesterol.

When your doctor states that your cholesterol is 250 mg (6.5 mmol), he or she is giving you the total amount of cholesterol in your blood, which includes LDL cholesterol and HDL cholesterol. The total figure is not broken down unless specifically requested by the doctor. The values given in mg are the amount in each 100 ml of blood.

Low-Density Lipoprotein ("Bad") Cholesterol

The LDL is small and contains most of the cholesterol that is transported to cells. The higher the level of LDL cholesterol in the blood, the greater the risk of coronary heart disease; thus the term "bad" cholesterol. About 75 percent of the blood cholesterol is carried as LDL cholesterol.

High-Density Lipoprotein ("Good") Cholesterol

Much interest has been focused on HDL cholesterol, so called because it is very small in size and very high in density. It carries the cholesterol away from body cells such as the lining of arteries, thereby helping to keep the artery wall clean; thus the term "good" cholesterol. About 25 percent of the blood cholesterol is carried as HDL cholesterol. People with high levels of HDL cholesterol, greater than 60 mg (1.6 mmol), appear to live longer and have less coronary heart disease. People with levels less than 30 mg (0.8 mmol) have an increased risk of coronary heart disease. Do not be alarmed, however, if your HDL is less than 30 mg (.8 mmol). Not all individuals with low HDL levels get heart attacks. It is not clear why some people should have high and others very low values.

Most females and males prior to puberty have about the same cholesterol levels. Boys, however, at puberty have about a 20 percent drop in HDL and a rise in LDL cholesterol. The decrease in HDL cholesterol may be due to an increase in androgens. In men the HDL level stays fairly constant up to age 50, then starts to rise between 50 to 65. It is possible that this rise might be due to a decrease of androgens, which occurs during the male climacteric period, whereas in women there is a gradual rise in HDL cholesterol from age 25 onwards. Women are believed to be protected to post-menopause by this increase in HDL and by their hormonal status. Why women are protected from coronary heart disease until menopause and yet not protected from strokes is not easily explained, especially if atherosclerosis is the basis of both diseases.

There is a relationship between HDL cholesterol levels and population groups, foods, alcohol, exercise and drugs:

1. Population groups: The Japanese, Inuit men and the black population in England, Jamaica, South Africa and the United States appear to have higher HDL cholesterol levels than whites. The exact reason for this finding is unknown; it may be due to a combination of genetic or environmental factors and diet.

2. Foods: A low-saturated fat, low-cholesterol diet modified to be acceptable to patients does not cause a change in HDL cholesterol levels. However, a very low-saturated fat diet does cause a reduction in HDL cholesterol. A high-carbohydrate diet produces a mild fall in HDL cholesterol. A vegetarian diet may cause a slight decrease in HDL and this may be due to an increased carbohydrate intake. Obesity is associated with a low HDL level and patients with very high triglyceride levels and diabetics often have low HDL levels.

3. Exercise: Daily strenuous exercise such as long-distance running can increase HDL levels by 5 to 10 percent. It is unfortunate that moderate exercise five times weekly to produce the training effect (cardiovascular fitness) does not significantly increase HDL levels. No one has documented that a rise in HDL cholesterol from 40 to 45 mg reduces cardiovascular risk. There appears to be a clear difference between 30 and 50 mg with regards to risk. Therefore, we do not advise you to take up long-distance running to elevate your levels by 5 to 10 percent. Jogging one to three miles daily or every other day will produce the training effect but appears to have little or an inconsistent effect on HDL levels.

4. Drugs: There are a few drugs that alter HDL levels slightly; they are considered only experimental at this stage. Niacin causes a mild increase (5 to 15 percent) in HDL levels, but the drug causes too many adverse effects to justify its use. The pharmaceutical companies are certainly busy trying to

develop HDL-increasing compounds, but they will require several years of testing, especially with regards to safety. Small-dose estrogens are the safest and best regimen to increase HDL levels in women who are considered at risk.

A reasonable indication of the risk of coronary heart disease can be deduced from the amount of HDL cholesterol relative to the total cholesterol. For example, if your total cholesterol is 240 mg and HDL cholesterol 60 mg, the percent of HDL cholesterol will be $(60 \div 240) \times 100 = 25$ percent. This puts you into the below-average coronary heart disease risk (i.e., good risk). The risk categories are as follows:

Coronary Heart Disease Risk	Percent HDL Cholesterol
Lowest risk group	Greater than 28
Below average	22-28
Average	15-22
High	7-15
Highest	Less than 7

Very-Low-Density Lipoprotein (VLDL)

The VLDL is very large and low in density. VLDL transports triglycerides, which are used mainly as a fuel; for example, in exercising muscle. The evidence linking elevated blood triglyceride levels with coronary heart disease is very weak and unclear. Thus, an elevated blood triglyceride level alone is not of importance. Weight reduction or cessation of alcohol intake always causes a marked reduction in triglyceride levels but does not alter LDL cholesterol levels.

GENETIC DEFECT AND CHOLESTEROL

In very rare cases, marked elevation of cholesterol (600 to 1,200 mg) is caused by a genetic defect. A receptor on the surface of cells (LDL receptors) removes LDL cholesterol from the blood. These receptors are genetically deficient in approximately one in 1,000 Americans and cause a marked increase in blood cholesterol. Deposits of cholesterol (xanthomas) occur as creamy yellow streaks under the skin eyelids, or on the Achilles tendon, the back of the hands and over bony prominences such as the knees and elbows. These people may have coronary heart disease in childhood or early adult life, but fortunately, the condition is very rare. Racial differences may determine the number of LDL receptors, and thus the ability to remove LDL cholesterol gradually from the blood stream is affected.

About 20 percent of the population have all the luck. They can eat a high-cholesterol, saturated-fat diet and violate all rules yet never get significant coronary heart disease and live beyond 79.

BLOOD TESTS

The blood cholesterol measurement gives the total blood cholesterol, i.e., LDL cholesterol plus HDL cholesterol. The food you eat does not have an immediate effect on your total blood cholesterol and HDL cholesterol measurements, so fasting is not necessary for their determination. Triglyceride level is not an independent risk factor and therefore widespread screening for elevated triglycerides is not warranted. It is also an expensive investigation. If your doctor thinks that triglyceride determination is necessary, you must fast for 14 hours before blood is taken. Blood tests for glucose, diabetes and triglycerides are the only tests for which it is necessary to fast for 12 to 14 hours before the test.

Determination of LDL cholesterol is not done routinely, because it is a difficult, time-consuming and expensive technique. It must be done fasting because it is calculated by a formula that requires a triglyceride blood level, which can only be done after fasting 12 hours. If the total cholesterol is less that 190 mg (4.9 mmol) and the HDL is greater than 39 mg (1 mmol), there is no need to worry about your LDL. If the total cholesterol is greater than 240 mg (6.2 mmol) and the HDL is less than 39 mg (1 mmol), the LDL levels should be estimated. If you have coronary heart disease, the level of LDL is of paramount importance and should be maintained at less than 100 mg (2.6 mmol).

SATURATED FATS

All animal fat is saturated and solid at normal room temperatures. The degree of hydrogenation of a fat determines how solid and saturated it is. Saturated fats are broken down in the body and increase blood cholesterol. Therefore, the most effective dietary method of lowering blood cholesterol is to reduce your intake of saturated fats. High-cholesterol foods are few, therefore we do not use the term low-cholesterol diet.

Vegetable fats are unsaturated and almost all are liquid at room temperatures. There are three vegetable oils that you must avoid: *coconut oil, palm oil and peanut oil.* Coconut oil contains a high amount of saturated fat and is commonly used for cooking in several countries. It is also used in North America in nondairy cream substitutes, for example, coffee cream. Therefore, *beware of coffee cream substitutes.* Palm oil contains significant amounts of saturated fat, and peanut oil, though mainly unsaturated, has certain fatty acids that produce plaques of atheroma in animals. The only vegetable that contains a little saturated fat is the avocado; therefore, low-cholesterol, low-fat diets, often recommend that you avoid avocados. You will note from Table 1, however, that although a large avocado contains a significant amount of fat, only a little of it is saturated, and no cholesterol is present. Therefore, one avocado a week is an excellent food, especially if a high potassium intake is required.

POLYUNSATURATES AND LINOLENIC ACID

The replacement of some saturated fats in the diet by polyunsaturated, monounsaturated and other unsaturated fats found in abundance in vegetable oil reduces blood LDL (bad) cholesterol. The saturated and polyunsaturated fat content of commonly used foods are given in Table 1.

Oils recommended for the preparation of meals include: canola, olive and soybean because they contain alpha-linolenic acid, very low cholesterol and minimum of saturated fat; for example, "cholesterol-free" canola oil contains 6 percent saturates and will produce a small amount of cholesterol in the body. Not all vegetable oils claim to be cholesterol free but contain significant saturated fats. Margarine made with these oils, hydrogenated or nonhydrogenated, are suitable (see Hydrogenated Fats), but because margarines contain a small amount of saturated fat and hydrogenation remains controversial, they should be used in moderation. Some products may have palm or coconut oil added to enhance hardening; these two oils are not recommended (see

Table 1). Olive oil is recommended for salads, but olive oil margarines may contain palm oil to enhance hardening. Thus you need to read labels carefully. Some margarines claim that they contain no cholesterol and are nonhydrogenated yet they contain palm oil.

It is important to note that many recipes developed for weight reduction diets tend to cut out carbohydrate foods in order to decrease weight and may even introduce foods that increase blood clotting and cholesterol. Therefore, be careful in choosing "popular" weight reduction diets. Consult Table 1 and the instructions given under Heart Attack Prevention Diet.

CHOLESTEROL AND DIETS

Diets to reduce atherosclerosis or heart attacks must be tailored to meet the needs of the individual, since each family has different eating habits. We emphasize that special recipes and diet sheets may be misleading, and difficult to follow for a lifetime. Therefore, we do not recommend recipes or diet sheets in this book. Any person requiring a diet may consult Table 1, or similar information.

It is recommended that you use foods that contain a low amount of saturated fat and cholesterol, and make an effort to increase your intake of polyunsaturated and monounsaturated fat, linolenic acid and foods that have a favorable effect on blood clotting (see Blood Clots). Reduction in the intake of cholesterol alone is not sufficient since saturated fat is converted into cholesterol in the body. Therefore, you must reduce your saturated fat intake. The recommendation made by the American Heart Association and followed by many Americans is as follows:

Total fat intake should be reduced from the average 40 percent of calories to 30 percent. Polyunsaturated fat should provide up to 10 percent of calories and the polyunsaturated fat to saturated fat (P/S) ratio should be about 1:1. Carbohydrate intake should be increased from an average of about 45 percent to 55 percent to maintain average body weight, and protein intake should remain at about 12 to 14 percent. It is believed that reducing dietary fat intake as well as stopping smoking by many individuals has provided a decline in the incidence of coronary heart disease mortality.

TABLE 1   **Saturated Fat, Polyunsaturated and Cholesterol Content of Foods**

ITEM*	Cholesterol	Total Fat	Saturated Fat	Not Recom.	Recom.**	Use Sparingly
	mg	g	g			
MEATS						
beef liver	395	10	3	X		
kidney	725	11	4	X		
sweetbread	420	21	—	X		
lean beef	82	5	2		●●	
roast beef						
rib	85	33	14	X		●
rump	85	21	9	X		
stewing	82	27	11	X		●
lean	82	9	4		●●	
ground	85	18	8	X		●
steak						
sirloin	85	25	10	X		●
lean	85	5	2		●●	
veal	90	12	5		●●	
lamb						
lean	90	7	4			●
chop & fat	110	33	18	X		
ham						
fat roasted	80	28	7	X		
boiled, sliced	80	18	5			●
pork chop	80	30	12	X		
chicken						
breast						
and skin	72	6	1		●●	
drumstick						
fried	80	9	2		●●	
turkey	80	5	2		●●	
FISH						
sole	45	1	trace		●●	
trout	50	13	3		●●	
tuna	60	7	2		●●	

*   Quantity is 3 oz, 90 g unless specified, 15 ml = one tablespoon.

**   Foods recommended contain less than 5 g saturated fat per 3 oz.

TABLE 1 cont'd	Saturated Fat, Polyunsaturated and Cholesterol Content of Foods					
ITEM*	Cholesterol	Total Fat	Saturated Fat	Not Recom.	Recom.**	Use Sparingly
	mg	g	g			
salmon						
fresh	42	7	1		••	
canned	32	11	2		••	
mackerel	85	10	2		••	
halibut	54	6	trace		••	
crabmeat	91	1	trace			•
shrimps	130	1	trace			•
lobster 450 g	80	1	trace			•
butter 30 ml	60	25	16	X		
egg 50 g	275	6	2		••	
substitute	0	0	0		••	
buttermilk†	10	2	1			
yogurt†						
250 ml	16	3	2		••	

ITEM*	Cholesterol	Total Fat	Saturated Fat	Polyunsat- urated	Not Recom.	Recom.**	Use Sparingly
	mg	g	g				
whole milk							
250 ml	35	9	5				•
2%	20	5	3			••	
skim milk	trace	trace	trace			••	
avocados							
1/3 California	0	11	2			••	
1/3 Florida	0	6.5	1			••	
ice cream							
125 ml							
vanilla, reg.	32	8	5				•
125 ml rich	46	12	8		X		

* Quantity is 3 oz, 90 g unless specified, 15 ml = one tablespoon.
** Foods recommended contain less than 5 g saturated fat per 3 oz.
† Low-fat milk, 2%.

ITEM*	Cholesterol	Total Fat	Saturated Fat	Polyunsat-urated	Not Recom.	Recom.**	Use Sparingly
	mg	g	g				
butter	30	11	7	trace			●
lard	12	13	5	1	X		
OILS							
canola	0	14	.5	8		●●	
corn oil	0	14	1	7		●●	
rapeseed	0	14	1	3	X		
safflower	0	13	1	10		●●	
sunflower	0	14	1	9		●●	
soybean	0	14	2	7		●●	
coconut	0	14	12	.2	X		
palm	0		7	.2	X		
olive	0	14	2	1		●●	
peanut		14	2	4	X		
cheese 1 oz							
brick	27	8	6	trace			●
blue	24			trace		●●	
cheddar	30	10	6	trace			●
cottage†	2	.6	.5	trace		●●	
skim milk							
processed	0	trace	trace	trace		●●	
NUTS 1 oz 30 g							
almonds	0	16	1	3		●●	
brazil nuts	0	22	5	8	X		
cashews	0	13	3	2	X		
coconut	0	13	11	trace	X		
peanuts	0	17	3	4	X		
peanut butter	0	7.5	1.5	2	X		
pecans	0	21	2	5			●
walnuts	0	19	2	11		●●	

TABLE 1 cont'd — Saturated Fat, Polyunsaturated and Cholesterol Content of Foods

*   Quantity is 3 oz, 90 g unless specified, 15 ml = one tablespoon.
** Foods recommended contain less than 5 g saturated fat per 3 oz.
†   Low-fat milk, 2%.

The United Kingdom has not shared, however, in the slight decline in mortality that has been experienced in Australia, Belgium, Canada, Finland, Norway and the United States. Scotland has moved up in the world league of coronary deaths to second for men and first for women, and Northern Ireland has moved to third for men and second for women. In the United Kingdom, fat intake has remained the same for the past 30 years at about 40 percent of food energy and even increased between 1974 and 1982 to 41 percent of food energy. Consequently in mid-1984, the Department of Health and Social Security made the following recommendations to physicians and the general public in the United Kingdom: Reduce the total fat intake to 35 percent of food energy, with saturated fats making up no more than 11 percent. Increase the polyunsaturated to saturated ratio from the present 0.27 to about 0.45. The intake of polyunsaturated acids presently at 5 percent of food energy should reach 7 percent, which is less than the American and World Health Organization's suggestion of 10 percent. The U.K. panel claims that the effects on the population of a P/S ratio of 1.0 and beyond are unknown. Individuals who are considered to have a high risk of developing coronary heart disease are advised to cut fats to 30 percent of food energy, with saturated fats contributing no more than 10 percent, i.e., identical to the recommendation in the United States. Thus there is consensus on both sides of the Atlantic. (See Heart Attack Prevention Diet.)

CHOLESTEROL-LOWERING DRUGS

HMG-CoA Reductase Inhibitors (Statins)

The statins: fluvastatin, lovastatin, pravastatin and simvastatin are new cholesterol-lowering agents that are effective and have few side effects. They cause a 15 to 30 percent reduction in total, or LDL (bad), cholesterol. They may cause a small, 1 to 8 percent, increase in HDL (good) cholesterol, but this effect is variable. Clinical trials have shown that these agents decrease LDL cholesterol levels and reduce the risk of heart attack and death from heart attacks (see Cholesterol).

Mild side effects include: headaches, ache in muscles, pain in the upper abdomen, but they do not cause gastritis, ulcers or bleeding. An increase in the liver enzymes may be detected on blood test, but the risk subsides on stopping the drug. **Caution:** do not take with niacin or fibrates: gemfibrozil, fenofibrate; contraindicated in pregnancy.

Fluvastatin (Lescol)

Supplied: Capsules: 20 mg.
Dosage: 20 to 40 mg after the evening meal or bedtime.

Lovastatin (Mevacor)

Supplied: Tablets: 10, 20, 40 mg.
Dosage: 10 to 40 mg after the evening meal.

Pravastatin (Pravachol)

Supplied: Tablets: 10, 20 mg.
Dosage: 10 to 40 mg after the evening meal or bedtime.

Simvastatin (Zocor)

Supplied: Tablets: 5, 10, 20 mg.
Dosage: 10 to 40 mg after the evening meal.

Cholestyramine (Questran)

Supplied: Powder in packets or in cans with a scoop.
Dosage: 12 to 24 grams (g) daily in liquid a half hour before to a half hour after meals. Start with 4 g (one scoop) twice daily for one week, then 4 g three times daily for one month and if necessary thereafter increase to 8 g three times daily.

Cholestyramine and colestipol are not absorbed from the gut and act by binding bile salts in the intestine. This action causes the liver to increase the conversion of cholesterol to bile acids, which are excreted in the bile. These agents are useful when combined with statins in patients with blood cholesterol greater than 360 mg (9 mmol).

The drug has no serious side effects. Constipation, nausea, bloating, gas and abdominal cramps may occur. High doses taken for several years can cause poor absorption of certain vitamins. The drugs may interfere with the absorption of digoxin and blood thinners (anticoagulants). Palatability is improved by mixing the product with fruit juice. Your doctor will decide when to use this potentially useful drug. Usually the patient is under age 55, and the blood cholesterol is greater than 260 mg (6.7 mmol) despite a six-month trial of diet.

Colestipol

Supplied: Powder.
Dosage: 12 to 30 g daily in liquid taken a half hour before to a half hour after meals and four hours apart from other medications.

Colestipol is a resin similar to cholestyramine with similar side effects but better patient acceptance.

Gemfibrozil

Supplied: Capsules: 300 mg (store below 86°F, 30°C).
Dosage: 300 mg taken about a half hour before the morning and the evening meal for one to two weeks, then 600 mg twice daily.

Gemfibrozil causes a 5 to 10 percent reduction in serum cholesterol, 30 to 40 percent reduction in triglycerides and a significant increase in HDL ("good") cholesterol. Side effects include stomach pain and bloating in less than 5 percent of patients. Gall stones may occur.

Niacin (Nicotinic Acid)

This drug is not often used because of prominent side effects, which include flushing, itching, nausea, abdominal pain, diarrhea, jaundice, gout, palpitations and increased blood sugar in diabetics. The drug should not be used if you have low blood pressure or a heart attack, heart failure, liver disease, a stomach ulcer or diabetes. It is not advisable to combine niacin with statins because severe damage to muscles and the kidneys may occur.

PREVENTION STRATEGY

If you are age 20 to 70, it is advisable to know your total blood cholesterol and HDL ("good") cholesterol. If the values are optimal at age 25 to 30, testing can be repeated every five years, and it won't change too much. To do otherwise will strain the finances of people and the state for very little return.

The answer to the question "Is lowering cholesterol important?" is yes. The evidence is clear. If you can decrease your blood cholesterol to less than 190 mg (4.8 mmol), and LDL cholesterol to less than 120 mg (3 mmol), you can substantially decrease risk of having a heart attack. More than 33 percent of the North American population age 40 to 60 have cholesterol levels in the borderline range of 210 to 240 mg, and it is in this group that the majority of heart attacks occur. They have, therefore, a cholesterol level that maybe accepted as normal or borderline by their doctor, but is clearly abnormal because it causes a high risk of coronary heart disease. We are in agreement with the experts who are concerned with this large population group, and strongly advise you to lower your so-called "borderline cholesterol," which is actually undesirably high. Patients with angina or a heart attack should maintain their LDL cholesterol level at less than 100 mg (2.6 mmol).

CONGENITAL HEART DISEASE

Congenital heart disease is a general term that refers to defects of the heart that occur during the development of the fetus. They are present at birth but may be discovered much later.

The exact causes of congenital heart disease, which occurs in about 0.8 percent of live births, is unknown. Approximately 10 percent of all congenital cardiac defects can be accounted for by chromosomal aberrations or genetic mutations or transmission. Down's syndrome is the most common chromosome aberration and occurs in about one in every 700 births; the risk rises steeply if the mother is above age 35 and is as high as 4 percent for women over age 44. In this condition, an atrial septal defect (ASD), a hole in the septum dividing the top chambers of the heart, occurs commonly.

Congenital defects associated with prenatal exposure to teratogens, which adversely affect embryonic or fetal development, include: infectious vectors such as rubella, radiation, drugs and chemicals including ACE inhibitors, alcohol, hydantoin, lithium, phenylalanine, thalidomide, trimethadione, valporic acid, vitamin D, anticoagulants and others. Because so little is known about the causes of the majority of congenital heart defects, and teratogens are strongly implicated in many, it must be emphasized that no medication should be taken during the first six months of pregnancy without prior consultation of a knowledgeable physician.

CONGENITAL CYANOTIC HEART DISEASE

Some babies born with congenital heart defects may appear blue at birth or during early childhood. During exertion and exercise, some children may become blue (cyanotic). In severe cases, the child is blue even at rest and the ends of the fingers appear club-like (finger clubbing). This form of congenital heart disease is called congenital cyanotic heart disease and is caused by blood which is deoxygenated flowing from the right side of the heart to the left side. It is usually caused by a hole in the heart combined with an obstruction to blood flow through one of the valves.

FALLOT'S TETRALOGY

Several defects are involved in this condition:

- A ventricular septal defect (VSD), a hole in the septum between the two ventricles.
- Right ventricular outflow obstruction in the area of the pulmonary valve. This causes hypertrophy of the right ventricle and a higher pressure in the right ventricle. Thus, deoxygenated blood flows through the hole in the heart from the right to the left ventricle. This deoxygenated, or blue, blood is pumped from the left ventricle into the arteries and general circulation. A blue discoloration is imparted to the lips, tongue, earlobes and other areas.
- Dextraposed aorta, overriding the septal defect.

Other anomalies, such as an atrial septal defect (ASD), VSD or patent ductus, can cause a right to left shunt and cyanotic problems if they are associated with pulmonary hypertension and enlargement of the right ventricle that markedly increase the right ventricular pressures.

The majority of congenital heart defects, however, result in blood flow from the left side of the heart carrying oxygenated blood into the right side and thus no bluish discoloration is observed. These children may have a completely normal childhood, and the defect is discovered in adolescence or young adulthood. In both congenital cyanotic heart disease and non-cyanotic heart disease, if the defects are large enough, children may show stunting of growth and are predisposed to frequent chest infections.

VENTRICULAR SEPTAL DEFECT (VSD)

Ventricular septal defect is the commonest congenital heart defect and occurs in up to 30 percent of cases. In children with a VSD there is a hole in the left ventricle that allows the blood to pass from the left to the right side. These conditions may be minor and allow patients to live beyond age 30 before a diagnosis is made. In many children with small VSDs, the defect closes naturally during the first 10 years of life. When the VSD is large and causes shortness of breath, the defect can be closed surgically.

ATRIAL SEPTAL DEFECT (ASD)

The second commonest defect is a hole in the septum between the top chambers of the heart, atrial septal defect. Patients may tolerate this defect for several years, and some are asymptomatic until after age 35. The defect causing ASD is easily closed surgically, but in recent years, the defect has been patched using a nonsurgical technique.

PATENT DUCTUS ARTERIOSUS

During fetal life, blood flows from the pulmonary artery into the aorta through a short connecting duct (ductus arteriosus). After birth, sudden expansion of the lungs and tying of the umbilical chord cause changes in the pressures and oxygen content in the duct, which constricts and closes during the first few days of life.

The duct can remain patent in some children, particularly in premature infants. A patent ductus is a common congenital lesion and usually causes a left to right shunt. Oxygenated blood flows from the aorta to the pulmonary artery to reach the lungs. A large shunt over several years may cause hypertension in the pulmonary circulation and lead to cyanotic heart disease. Surgical division or occlusion of the ductus is not a difficult operation. A nonsurgical approach is being investigated and involves the use of a polyurethane foam umbrella, which is introduced via a vein and finally plugs the duct. Results of this procedure are encouraging.

PULMONARY VALVE STENOSIS

The valve is narrowed (stenosis), thus the right ventricle has difficulty ejecting blood into the lungs across the pulmonary valve (see Fig. 11). The nonsurgical therapy includes balloon valvuloplasty. Balloon dilatation catheters are advanced through the femoral vein and when in position across the tight pulmonary valve, the balloon is inflated. Over the past 12 years, this technique has given excellent and lasting results with minimal risk.

COARCTATION OF THE AORTA

Coarctation of the aorta is a congenital narrowing of the aorta as the artery winds its way from the top of the heart (see Fig. 11). The condition may be discovered when the child is an infant if the coarctation is severe or if an astute physician correctly interprets the signs. Some 80 percent of children, however, have a mild coarctation or develop an extensive corollary system of vessels that carry blood past the coarct and such children may have no symptoms until they reach adolescence; some children have no symptoms until they reach the age of 15 to 30.

Early diagnosis is essential to ensure timely surgical or nonsurgical correction. Although there are remarkably specific physical signs that make diagnosis straightforward in the doctor's office, it is one of the most commonly overlooked diagnoses in children. A diagnosis can be made within minutes if the physician feels the femoral pulses and finds them absent or weak. Also, there is accompanying high blood pressure in the arms and low pressure in the legs. More than 80 percent of coarctations are situated just beyond the ductus arteriosus and, fortunately, beyond the beginning of the left subclavian artery, which supplies blood to the left upper limb.

Because the aorta is constricted, the limbs are blood starved. There is hypertension in the upper part of the body and the blood pressure is low in the legs. Symptoms result from:

- Lack of adequate blood supply to the lower limbs, causing coldness, numbness, heaviness of the legs and feet, pain in the muscle, intermittent claudication and leg cramps.
- Dizziness, headaches, nosebleeds, shortness of breath and palpitations.
- Complications include: angina, heart failure, aortic rupture and cerebral hemorrhage, particularly from associated berry aneurysms at the base of the brain. All patients should be screened to exclude berry aneurysms, polycystic kidney and bicuspid aortic valve. Endocarditis of a bicuspid valve or the aorta in the arch or just distal to the coarctation may occur.

Treatment is best achieved with surgery. Balloon dilatation is recommended for recurrent coarctation and has had a success rate of about 80 percent. Results of the Valvuloplasty and Angioplasty of Congenital Anomalies Registry indicate a success rate that is comparable with surgery for recurrent coarctation. As first-step therapy, however, balloon dilatation is considered investigational. Protection from a rupture during the procedure is of concern because the coarctation area is not surrounded by scar tissue as occurs after surgery. Because dilatation of the artery causes tears in the wall (intima and media), long-term follow-up is required to exclude the possibility of aneurysm formation. Continued evaluation and long-term assessment are necessary before the procedure can be considered first choice.

After correction of the coarctation, the blood pressure may increase over the ensuing years. Thus close follow-up is necessary. Because constriction of the aorta causes reduced blood flow to the kidney, the renin angiotensin system is stimulated and this increases blood pressure. ACE inhibitors constitute rational therapy for the management of hypertension but are not always successful.

CORONARY ARTERIES

The *coronary arteries* run along the outer surface of the heart (see Fig. 2). There are two main coronary arteries, left and right, which originate at the root of the aorta as it leaves the heart. The left main coronary artery is very short, 0.1 to 4 centimeters, and divides almost immediately into two branches. The first branch, called the anterior descending artery, runs down the front or anterior surface of the heart, near the undersurface of the left margin of the breastbone. It supplies blood to a major portion of the left ventricle. The second branch, called the circumflex artery, circles around and feeds the back of the heart. The right coronary artery leaves the aorta, veers sharply left, then is directed toward the breastbone and curves downward to run along the border of the right ventricle. The right coronary artery supplies branches to the electrical system, which involves special cells that cause the heart to beat (the sinus node pacemaker), and to the conducting bridge for electrical transmission between the atrium and ventricle (atrioventricular node). The branches subdivide several times and perforate the heart muscle at different points to bring nutrients to the muscle. These arteries have nothing to do with the blood flow inside the heart, which is pumped around the body. In addition, their internal diameter is only about the size of a soda straw.

You can consider the heart as being supplied by four arteries: the left main coronary artery, the left anterior descending, the circumflex, and the right coronary arteries. It is easy to visualize blockage of the left main coronary artery as the most dangerous, as it would block off two major arteries. Fortunately, this is rare. Most heart attacks are due to blocks in the right coronary artery, the anterior descending, and less commonly, the circumflex, or smaller branches of these three arteries (see Fig. 1).

Blockage of the coronary arteries by atherosclerosis is extremely common and more than 50 percent of North American males over age 35 and females over age 50 have significant plaques of atheroma partially obstructing one or more coronary arteries. These partially obstructing plaques of atheroma jut into the lumen of the artery and disturb the free flow of blood to the heart muscle. The plaques do not usually cause symptoms, but in some individuals, chest pain (angina) occurs on exertion because the partially obstructed artery cannot supply enough blood and oxygen during exertion (see Figs. 1 and 3). For more information on angina, see Angina.

CORONARY ARTERY BYPASS SURGERY

Dr. Rene Favoloro of Argentina performed the first coronary artery bypass graft (CABG) in 1967 at the Cleveland Clinic. He used a vein from a patient's leg to bypass the obstruction in the coronary artery. Since that time, several million bypass operations have been performed. The procedure is a simple one: A vein from the patient's leg is removed and inserted into the aorta as it leaves the heart; the other end of the vein is joined to the coronary artery below the blockage. Blood then flows from the aorta through the vein graft beyond the blockage to the coronary artery and to the heart muscle (see Fig. 10). When possible, surgeons prefer to use the internal mammary artery instead of using a vein graft to bypass the blockage in the important left anterior descending artery (see Figs. 2 and 10).

Indications

If angina is not adequately relieved by the combination of a beta-blocker, a nitrate and a calcium blocker and lifestyle is deemed unacceptable by the patient or the physician, coronary artery bypass surgery is usually recommended. The main aim of surgery is therefore to relieve pain. The complete relief of pain is certainly most satisfying and this is achieved in 90 percent of patients, whereas drugs achieve this goal in less than 50 percent. Drugs lessen the frequency of angina by about 60 percent in approximately 60 percent of patients treated. Such patients are satisfied and surgery is not indicated. Thus about 20 percent of patients with angina are not satisfactorily controlled. Half of these are elderly or have illness that contraindicate surgical intervention. Thus about 10 out of every 100 patients with "stable" angina are recommended to have coronary arteriography with a view to coronary bypass surgery. In some surgical centers, indications are broadened and many more patients are selected for surgery. The majority of patients with unstable angina

CORONARY BYPASS GRAFT
Blood flows from the aorta to a coronary artery bypassing the blockage

FIGURE 10

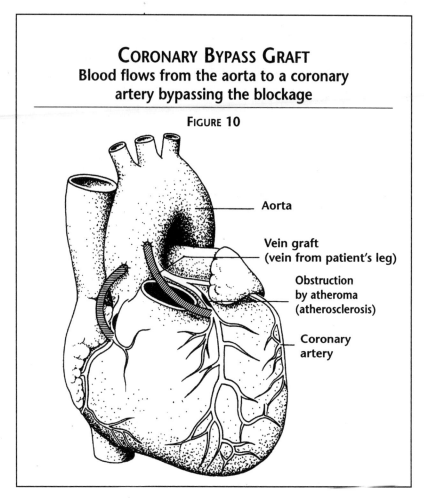

Aorta

Vein graft
(vein from patient's leg)

Obstruction
by atheroma
(atherosclerosis)

Coronary
artery

should be offered surgery if no major contraindication exists. Patients up to age 80 and, in some places, over age 80, are offered surgery. When surgery is done in 100 patients, the statistical outcome is as follows: The risk of dying during the surgery or within three days is 1 to 2 percent. Approximately 10 percent of patients have a heart attack during surgery, although it is usually silent and recovery is the rule. Approximately 90 patients get complete relief for two or more years. At the end of two years, 15 to 18 patients have obstruction of their grafts and some of these get a recurrence of the angina. Presently, with the addition of medication such as aspirin, fewer grafts become blocked. After five years, about 70 percent of patients are still pain-free, lead active lives, and enjoy life to the fullest — a situation that does not materialize with the use of drug treatment in patients with frequent episodes of angina.

Bypass surgery is simple to perform and there are few complications. Cardiac surgeons can be proud of this operation, which provides major relief for suffering and can prolong life in a selected few. We can visualize many successful operations using angioplasty and laser therapy during the next 20 years, but unless atherosclerosis is prevented, and this seems to be out of reach for the next 50 years, coronary artery bypass surgery will play a substantial role for longer than some experts predict.

Patients who have had surgery must understand that the other arteries and points in the coronary artery below the graft can develop further atherosclerosis since the operation does not cure the disease. In addition, a blood clot (coronary thrombosis) can form in any individual at any time without warning. Therefore, coronary bypass surgery does not prevent a second or third heart attack although it may prevent death in a few.

Approximately 50 percent of the grafts become blocked after 10 years, particularly in patients who smoke, or have hypertension, diabetes or an LDL cholesterol level greater than 120 mg (3 mmol).

Prolongation of life may be achieved in patients with stable or unstable angina and serious blockage of arteries in the following types:

1. Individuals who have severe narrowing of the left main coronary artery before it divides. This is the anatomical lesion for which surgery is universally accepted and is fortunately rare.
2. Individuals who have triple vessel disease, that is, severe obstruction of the right coronary, the left anterior descending and the circumflex arteries, especially in patients with decreased function of the left ventricular muscle. The ejection fraction (EF), the amount of blood the ventricle puts out into the aorta with each beat, is an important measure of the strength of the heart muscle. The value is expressed as a percentage. Normal EF is more than 50 percent. An EF of less than 40 percent carries a bad prognosis and less than 25 percent a very poor prognosis. Surgery is highly beneficial in patients with an EF between 25 and 45 percent.
3. If the left anterior descending artery is blocked before its first branch, plus two other vessels have more than 80 percent obstruction and angioplasty is not possible.

Some clinical trials indicate that prolongation of life may be achieved in the above types of patients. We concur with these results although there are some reports to the contrary.

Contraindications

Severe damage to the heart muscle as manifested by recurrent heart failure unresponsive to aggressive medical therapy and an ejection fraction of less than 25 percent is a major contraindication. Such patients are very short of breath and often have fluid in the lungs. Shortness of breath cannot be relieved by surgery, and the heart muscle is not strengthened. Several heart attacks cause large areas of scarring, and the scar tissue is very weak. Scar tissue is dead and not supplied with blood; therefore, a bypass graft does not feed blood to that area. Heart failure in the presence of an acute heart attack that clears within the first seven days is not a contraindication to bypass surgery several months later because the heart muscle recovers more than 75 percent of its function; this recovery may prevail for more than 25 years.

Maintenance medications that are given after coronary bypass surgery include: 325 mg of aspirin (coated) daily.

Drugs such as oral nitrates and calcium antagonists are not usually required except in a few patients if angina recurs. Many patients are continued for years on these unproven and costly drugs. Beta-blockers may be given because *they prolong life.*

Patients are strongly advised not to recommence smoking. They are encouraged to engage in an exercise program and maintain a low-cholesterol-low-saturated-fat diet. The blood pressure should be checked every four months to be sure that it is not elevated since this may aggravate the problems of blockage in the graft.

It is important to understand that atherosclerotic disease is not cured by surgery. Coronary thrombosis can still occur. The vein graft can develop atherosclerosis over a period of 10 to 15 years as veins are not usually subjected to the blood pressure found in arteries. The average pressure found within veins is normally about 5 to 7 mm Hg as compared to the normal pressure in arteries of about 110 to 150 mm Hg. One study showed that 10 years post surgery, more than half of the grafts were narrowed or blocked — particularly in individuals who continued to smoke cigarettes or in those with hypertension and increased cholesterol levels. Clinical trials done in 1994 to 1995 have established that the use of statins to maintain LDL cholesterol at less than 100 mg (2.5 mmol) prevents the progression of atheroma and reduces the need for angioplasty and repeat bypass surgery (see Cholesterol).

CORONARY HEART (ARTERY) DISEASE

When the coronary arteries are partially blocked by atherosclerosis so as to cause symptoms, many doctors use the term atherosclerotic heart disease or ischemic heart disease. Others use the term coronary heart disease, because it is the coronary arteries that are affected. Because the term coronary heart disease is easier to understand, this term is used throughout the book. Angina and heart attacks are the two main manifestations of coronary heart disease. See sections on Angina, Heart Attacks, Atherosclerosis/ Atheroma and Figs. 1 and 3.

COUGH AND COLD REMEDIES

Remedies advertised for the management of stubborn coughs and colds commonly contain one of the following:

- Dextromethorphan: A cough suppressant that is effective in patients with dry, hacking, bothersome cough.
- Codeine: A weak cough suppressant that can cause undesirable effects such as dizziness, nausea and constipation.
- Guaiphenesin: An expectorant that is claimed to liquify sputum. This agent has a weak effect; it is nearly impossible to liquify thick, tenacious phlegm. The majority of patients get no relief from the use of this compound.
- Antihistamine: A commonly used antihistamine is diphenhydramine. It is important to note that coughs and colds are not due to allergies, and antihistamines do not relieve symptoms. Antihistamines are commonly found in cough mixtures and may cause an increase in heart rate and drowsiness. The addition of an antihistamine to a cough mixture is an error that has been perpetuated by the pharmaceutical industry.
- Decongestants: These are stimulants that can cause an

increase in heart rate, palpitations and an increase in blood pressure. Decongestants should be avoided if you have high blood pressure, angina or heart attacks. Commonly used decongestants include ephedrine, pseudoephedrine, phenylephrine and phenylpropanolamine. Decongestants have no role in the management of cough. They provide only some symptomatic relief by decongesting nasal passages in patients with severe sinusitis or severe nasal congestion.

Patients with chronic bronchitis or emphysema and those suspected of having acute bronchitis or pneumonia should avoid using cough suppressants. Cough expectorants are of no value.

DENTAL WORK AND HEART DISEASE

Some individuals must take antibiotics before dental work to prevent infection of heart valves that are abnormal or artificial. Patients who have had angina or heart attacks or have angina and other types of heart disease do not require antibiotics for dental work. An infection of a heart valve is called endocarditis (see Bacterial Endocarditis under Valve Diseases). Patients with valves damaged by rheumatic fever, mitral valve prolapse and other forms of valve disease should take antibiotics one hour before and six hours after dental work (see Bacterial Endocarditis).

The current recommendations of the American Heart Association are as follows:

- For dental work, including hygienist treatment, and other surgical procedures that may cause bacteria to enter the bloodstream: patients should be given amoxicillin, 3 g one hour before and 1.5 g six hours later. Patients who are allergic to penicillin (amoxicillin) should take 300 mg (2 capsules of 150 mg) clindamycin one hour before and two hours after dental work. Clindamycin has replaced erythromycin in patients allergic to penicillin, or in those who have side effects from amoxicillin, because erythromycin causes abdominal cramps. Clindamycin may be used to replace amoxicillin because only four capsules are required versus nine for amoxicillin.

- Intravenous antibiotics should be given to high-risk patients who are undergoing dental work and most types of surgery except for cataracts. Such patients should be given amoxicillin and gentamycin IV one hour prior to surgery or dental work and six hours later.

All patients who have been informed by their doctors that they have a significant heart murmur caused by a slightly damaged heart valve should inform their dentist and should carry this information and a prescription for antibiotics. All patients with mechanical or bio-prosthetic heart valves require antibiotics for dental work and for most types of surgery and biopsies.

DEPRESSION

Patients with depression may be treated with tricyclic antidepressants, such as amitryptilline and imipramine derivatives. These drugs may cause an increase in heart rate. Some patients may feel the heart beats stronger and faster. Occasionally, serious abnormal heart rhythms may occur. These drugs must not be used concurrently with amiodarone or sotalol.

Fluoxetine and sertraline and similar agents must be used cautiously in patients with coronary heart disease; these drugs may cause angina attacks. Unexpected deaths have been reported, albeit rarely, with fluoxetine in patients with coronary heart disease and arrhythmias; a definite relationship has not been established. A few patients have been reported to have a very low concentration of sodium in the blood, particularly when taking diuretics.

DIABETES

Diabetes is a risk factor for the development of coronary heart disease: angina, heart attacks and heart failure. Diabetes usually causes an increases in LDL cholesterol, total cholesterol and triglycerides. Some diabetics experiencing a heart attack may complain of shortness of breath and weakness or nausea instead of chest pain.

There is no doubt that diabetes causes damage to arteries, especially the coronary, kidney and leg vessels. Diabetes affects 2 to 3 percent of the North American population. This 2 percent does not include individuals found to have mild elevation of blood sugar and those informed that they have a touch of diabetes or glucose intolerance. Mild glucose intolerance or possible mild chemical diabetes is not proven to carry the high risk of true diabetes. Many diabetics also have increased blood cholesterol and triglycerides. Atherosclerosis is common and is due to the combination of high cholesterol and damage to the arteries by the diabetic process.

Improved diet plans along with the techniques to achieve more efficient control of blood sugar may result in a reduction in cardiovascular complications. This hypothesis needs to be confirmed by further studies.

Diabetics with angina may not obtain maximum benefit from therapy with balloon angioplasty. Bypass surgery is often more effective.

DIGOXIN

Digoxin strengthens the heart muscle and causes more efficient pumping of blood. This drug has been used for over 200 years to treat the failing heart. When the heart muscle is weakened by different diseases and cannot pump blood adequately, patients experience severe shortness of breath and swelling of the legs; the condition is caused by heart failure. Digoxin is a mild drug, however, and is often used in combination with a diuretic, furosemide (see Digitalis in Heart Failure Drug Treatment).

DIURETICS

Diuretics, or "water pills," remove salt and water from the blood and eliminate these through the kidneys into the urine. Diuretics are commonly used to treat hypertension because an increase in sodium content of the blood and arteries causes blood pressure to rise (see Hypertension).

Diuretics are very important in the treatment of heart failure. They are more effective in relieving shortness of breath than digoxin or ACE inhibitors, the two other drugs used in combination to treat heart failure (see Heart Failure Drug Treatment). Diuretics used alone do not completely prevent the recurrence of heart failure and combination of the two or three agents is necessary.

EDEMA

Edema refers to a collection of liquid (fluid) under the skin. The liquid is composed of salt and water (brine). The fluid gravitates to the lowest or most dependent part of the body; thus edema is most prominent around ankles and feet. When salt and water retention is excessive, edema fluid may cause marked swelling of both legs to above the knees. The legs are brine-logged, not just waterlogged. Diuretics, which remove salt and water from the body, are used to relieve this condition. Marked edema occurs in heart failure, cirrhosis of the liver, some kidney diseases and when the albumin content of the blood is low.

Edema localized in one leg is not due to the conditions listed above but is usually caused by obstruction to veins in the leg or severe varicosities. Excessive heat may dilate veins in the legs, causing mild swelling of the feet. Some drugs such as calcium blockers and NSAIDs cause swelling of the ankles and feet.

ENDOCARDITIS

Endocarditis refers to infection of the valves in the heart. Normal valves have a very smooth, silky surface. Valves become swollen, rugged and rough when they have been affected by rheumatic fever or other conditions including mitral valve prolapse and bicuspid aortic valve. Rough or deformed valves may trap bacteria that occasionally gain entry to the blood, especially during dental and other surgical interventions (see Bacterial Endocarditis under Valve Diseases).

ETHANOL/ALCOHOL

Alcohol is a central nervous system and heart muscle depressant. In acute experiments, eight ounces of alcohol given to healthy students over a two-hour period decreased the amount of blood the heart pumped into the arteries (cardiac output) by 33 percent. Patients with enlarged hearts or previous heart failure should not take alcohol, since it decreases the force of heart muscle contraction and can cause heart failure.

High consumption of alcohol of any type, beer or liquor, for several years can cause a severe weakening of and damage to the heart muscle, and this leads to severe enlargement of the heart and heart failure (cardiomyopathy). Fortunately, the condition is rare. Low to moderate consumption of alcohol in healthy individuals or in patients with coronary heart disease without heart failure does not increase the risk of heart attack. Two to three ounces of alcohol daily can increase HDL cholesterol levels by 5 to 10 percent, but whether this modest rise can be protective is not proven and remains controversial.

BAD EFFECTS

Alcohol has three deleterious effects on the heart:

- Patients with a weak heart muscle causing heart failure with shortness of breath should discontinue alcohol. Alcohol will further weaken the heart muscle.
- Alcohol can cause abnormal heart rhythms in susceptible individuals. The heart beat becomes irregular due to the presence of premature beats. The irregularity may become bothersome, with a rapid irregular heart beat called atrial fibrillation (see Atrial Fibrillation). The occurrence of abnormal heart rhythms or palpitations may occur within hours of alcohol intake, but more commonly the disturbance occurs

12 to 24 hours after alcohol consumption.

- Excessive alcohol intake can cause direct damage to the heart muscle. Fortunately, this condition is rare. There appears to be a genetic predisposition to ethanol-induced heart muscle disease. Stretching of the heart muscle occurs and heart failure ensues. This condition becomes resistant to treatment and the prognosis is poor. Individuals with ethanol heart muscle disease commonly die within five years. If alcohol intake ceases, some patients recover with the help of special treatment. Fortunately, only the rare individual who has a genetic susceptibility develops heart muscle disease.

Alcohol has been associated with causing some rise in systolic blood pressure. Hypertensive individuals who consume more than two drinks daily may find that they require no drug treatment or minimal therapy for hypertension if alcohol intake is curtailed.

GOOD EFFECTS

One to two drinks daily over several years appears to cause a slight decrease in mortality from coronary heart disease. France has the second lowest coronary heart disease mortality rate and the highest alcohol intake despite an above-average dairy fat consumption. A lower coronary heart disease mortality in France is, however, associated with a high mortality rate from cirrhosis of the liver.

The evidence for greater protection against coronary heart disease by wine versus other alcoholic drinks is weak. Red wine may contain antioxidants and phenols, but their effect appears to be modest and some studies indicate that white wine is as beneficial as red. In a study in California, white wine appeared much more protective than red wine. A United States study of health professionals showed spirits to have the greatest beneficial effects. Thus there is no proof that wine is best and particularly there is no solid information that red wine is more protective. There is good evidence to support the notion that it is the ethanol content of beverages rather than antioxidants, phenols and chemicals that produces the beneficial effects. The effects of other components are modest.

Follow-up studies indicate that the maximum protection is obtained by consuming one or at most two drinks daily.

Consuming more than two drinks daily is associated with a high risk of mortality from cirrhosis.

Ethanol causes an increase in HDL (good) cholesterol, which is believed to be the explanation for the decrease of coronary heart disease mortality.

Ethanol consumption is not recommended by the medical profession as an adjunct to improve mortality of coronary heart disease. Alcohol does not protect from other forms of heart disease. The risk of death from cirrhosis of the liver increases in a population consuming more than four drinks daily; alcohol abuse has other undesirable effects. In addition, the possibility of genetic predisposition to alcoholism in several individuals is of concern. It is relevant, however, that individuals who are well disciplined and can limit their quota to one or at most two drinks daily may benefit from significant protection from coronary heart disease.

EXERCISE AND THE HEART

BENEFITS OF EXERCISE

One of the main reasons for practicing some form of regular, moderate exercise is that it always makes you feel and look better. Exercise does not have to be vigorous or strenuous to achieve important goals. Important psychological benefits can be produced by moderate exercise such as the combination of walking for 20 minutes, performing stretching exercises for 10 minutes, and where possible, cycling or swimming for 10 to 15 minutes daily or at least every second day. These simple exercises are practical, inexpensive and not time-consuming. In addition, such exercises pose no danger to individuals over the age of 40 and yet are sufficient to cause relaxation and produce a sense of well-being and a mental attitude that can better deal with stress.

If you do 30 to 40 minutes of moderate exercise a day, and add a favorite sport such as tennis, other racquet sports or skiing, you will attain a degree of fitness, i.e., you can be considered relatively fit. By "relatively fit," we mean that you have the stamina and energy to do your daily work and favorite sport without shortness of breath, muscle fatigue or a pounding heart.

Some people between the ages of 15 and 40, as well as 15 percent of North Americans over the age of 40, seek to exceed these achievements. Individuals who engage in regular vigorous exercise often reach a new "high," and studies have shown that high levels of endorphins are produced in the bodies of such individuals. Endorphins are opiate-like chemicals similar to morphine that increase pain threshold and euphoria. With regular vigorous exercise, cardiovascular conditioning is quickly achieved.

It is important to understand some of the terms that are used in describing various types of exercises:

Aerobic Exercise

Aerobic literally means "with air"; i.e., oxygen is required. Aerobic exercise involves the rhythmic contraction and relaxation of large muscle groups and movement of joints, for example, brisk walking, swimming, cycling, jogging and dancing.

Oxygen is obtained in the lungs and transported by the blood. Your exercising muscles require an increasing supply of oxygen, glucose and other constituents. The body gets the additional oxygen by increasing the rate of breathing, the heart rate and the output of blood from the heart. The amount of blood pumped each minute (cardiac output) increases from the average resting value of about five liters to around 20 liters. A large part of this output goes to the exercising muscles.

Aerobic exercises cause an increase in heart rate and systolic blood pressure; the diastolic blood pressure is unchanged or slightly increased. The blood flow through nonexercising muscles, the liver, intestine and kidneys, is reduced. If you exercise mainly your upper limbs, this will cause a slightly higher increase in heart rate and blood pressure than exercise utilizing the legs.

Isometric, or static, exercise

Isometric means "equal measure." The muscle fiber length remains the same when muscular tension is exerted against a fixed resistance; i.e., static exercise involves the development of tension within muscle fibers and results in little or no movement of bones and joints. Weightlifting, pushing against a wall, or waterskiing are examples. This type of exercise is generally not recommended for individuals who are over the age of 45 or who have hypertension or known heart disease, since it causes a marked increase in blood pressure during the effort. The pressure of tensed muscles squeezes blood vessels, and therefore, less blood passes through these arteries. Also, the constriction of blood vessels causes an increase in blood pressure. The heart works harder to pump against the resistance in the constricted arteries, but the amount of blood the heart pumps only increases slightly since the few muscles that are being used require less oxygen than would be required during isotonic exercise. Despite this lower oxygen requirement of the exercising muscle during static exercise, the heart work is increased and the heart muscle requires more oxygen. If coronary heart disease is present, the heart muscle may suffer from a shortage of oxygen that can result in chest pain or angina or precipitation of a heart attack. Hypertensive individuals must not engage in isometric exercises.

During static exercise there is an increased heart rate and blood pressure, but only a mild increase in cardiac output and rate of breathing. Therefore, physical conditioning may be achieved, but the cardiopulmonary conditioning training effect cannot be obtained.

Anaerobic Exercise

Anaerobic means "without oxygen," and energy is derived from the breakdown of glucose in the blood and muscle with the formation of lactic acid. Static exercise such as heavy weightlifting or very high intensity aerobic exercise such as a 100-yard sprint are examples of anaerobic exercise, and heart patients cannot take part in such exercises.

CARDIOVASCULAR CONDITIONING-TRAINING EFFECT

When a physically inactive individual suddenly decides to walk up four or five flights of stairs or commences unaccustomed aerobic exercise, he or she quickly gets winded or short of breath and feels the heart thumping away at a fast rate. The lack of physical fitness is obvious to the individual. If the same activity is repeated daily or every other day, after two or three weeks the individual no longer experiences the shortness of breath; heart rate increases only slightly and there is a faster return to normal resting heart rate after exercise; i.e., the training effect is achieved. Heart, lungs, blood vessels and muscles have started to adapt.

During exercise, muscles require an increase in oxygen supply. The lungs must take in more oxygen, the heart must pump faster and harder to get the oxygen to the muscles and the muscles must extract more oxygen.

The heart is a powerful muscular pump but needs oxygen to generate energy for its muscle contraction. The amount of oxygen the heart muscle requires at any time (myocardial oxygen consumption) can be determined by complicated techniques. A simple relationship, the product of the heart rate and systolic blood pressure, has been shown to be a reliable indicator of the heart muscle's oxygen requirement. Increased heart muscle efficiency is indicated by a decreased oxygen requirement for a similar amount of work. Regular exercise increases the efficiency of the heart muscle so that it requires less oxygen for the same amount of work. At rest, the heart muscle extracts about 65 percent of the oxygen reaching its muscle cells, and not much more can be extracted on exercise. Therefore, if the heart muscle requires more oxygen, the coronary arteries must dilate to supply more oxygenated blood. This situation can occur only if the coronary arteries are normal and capable of dilating.

With frequent exercise, the heart becomes conditioned to do the same work at a lower heart rate. You no longer feel your heart pumping away as if it wants to jump out of your chest or throat. If your exercise is then increased both in intensity and duration for at least 30 minutes daily, you will find that your resting heart rate may be reduced by five to 20 beats.

Your heart rate is controlled by the brain and nerves that innervate the heart and the pacemaker (sinus node). The nerves that stimulate the heart to beat faster are called "sympathetic nerves" and they are stimulated from the brain. For example, if someone is going to attack you and you wish to flee, the sympathetic nerves are stimulated by the fright, anxiety and tension. Noradrenaline produced by the nerve endings and adrenaline produced by the adrenal glands stimulate the heart to beat faster and stronger.

An opposing nerve called the vagus nerve (parasympathetic nerve) causes the heart to slow down. The "vagus nerve" is like the reins of a horse that keep the horse from running away out of control. Some individuals have an inborn, strong vagal nerve action and have a slow average resting heart rate that is about 64 instead of 72 beats per minute. Frequent exercise increases the effects of the vagal nerve (tightens the reins) and therefore leads to a slower heart rate. Many athletes have a resting heart rate of 35 to 50 beats per minute so that on exercise the heart rate goes up much less. In an untrained 50-year-old, a quarter-mile jog may produce a heart rate of 150 to 170 beats per minute. With training, the same exercise may cause a heart rate of only 120 to 140 beats per minute, and the product of heart rate and blood pressure will be reduced. It means that a conditioned heart will not have to work as hard to pump the same amount of blood. The heart muscle therefore requires less oxygen during the exercise.

The coronary arteries fill only when the heart muscle is relaxed (during diastole). A slower heart rate means that the heart is relaxed for a longer period of time and thus has more time to fill the normal or partially obstructed coronary arteries. Therefore, a better supply of oxygen and other nutrients reaches the heart muscle.

A fit heart idles at a lower speed and does not strain during maximal activity; i.e., the difference between the unfit and fit heart is similar to the performance of a poorly tuned 1934 car as opposed to a new 1996 model. We must caution that while frequent exercise may slightly lower your heart rate at rest and for a given exercise, medical experts agree that *there is no scientific evidence that this effect can prevent heart attacks*. The slower heart rate does not prevent clot formation or atherosclerosis.

During exercise the following important changes occur:

- The requirement for oxygen by exercising muscle causes a lack of oxygen. Therefore, the rate at which you breathe increases from about 12 breaths per minute to 24 to 30 per minute, so that more oxygen is taken into the lungs and given up to the blood.
- Resting muscles extract only about 30 percent of the oxygen from the blood bathing the muscle cells. Vigorously exercising muscle can extract over 75 percent of the circulating oxygen. The amount of oxygen extracted at peak exercise is your maximal oxygen uptake and reflects the limit of your endurance or cardiopulmonary (cardiovascular) conditioning. An increase in your maximal oxygen uptake is the adaptation of the body to aerobic exercise. The body makes more

efficient use of the oxygen available, and there is also less work for the heart. It is this physiological adaptation that allows you to have more stamina and less fatigue at a given level of aerobic exercise.

WEIGHT REDUCTION AND EXERCISE

A regular exercise program can cause mild weight reduction, which is greatly enhanced by a weight-reduction diet. Exercise is most helpful in long-term weight-reduction programs. Physical activity requires energy, which is measured in calories. Think of the body as having several factories. If you shut down half of these factories and let the other half work at half the speed, your output would be diminished. This is equivalent to turning down your metabolic rate (metabolic thermostat). If you go on a crash diet, your metabolic thermostat is turned down to get by on less food. Twenty to 40 minutes of aerobic exercise done regularly three to four times weekly can boost your metabolic rate by 20 to 30 percent, and this will accelerate the breakdown of fat stores. The body of an obese individual is programmed to form fat and to store it away. In addition, your cells slow down and you burn fewer calories than normal. Cells slow down even more if you are on a severe weight-reduction diet so as to conserve energy. The more you exercise, the more dependent you become on fat metabolism. Many obese individuals do not overeat, but their metabolic rate is so low that they store fat. Therefore, start exercising first, then a few weeks later start your diet and continue on an exercise program for at least one year to keep the weight down.

To burn 100 calories, a 170-pound individual needs to walk briskly 1 1/2 miles or jog one mile. Note that brisk walking is nearly as good as jogging since the speed at which you complete the distance makes little difference to the total amount of calories you burn. Therefore, a brisk mile in 15 minutes twice daily or two miles once daily is of value until you can add other exercises. If you do this daily, you will lose one pound in less than 14 days. If your diet usually provides 1,200 to 1,500 calories daily and you drop to a 1,000-calorie diet during this exercise program, you will have an additional one-pound loss in 14 days. This may seem small, but the good news is that in six months you will be 24 pounds lighter and you will be able to hold on to this reduction. Now that you are used to exercise, if you continue your program four days weekly, you will find it is easy to stay on a 1,000- to 1,200-calorie diet and you will maintain ideal weight. Exercise alone without restriction of calorie intake results in only mild weight reduction. Therefore, both exercise and diet should be used to achieve the best results.

EFFECTS ON BLOOD PRESSURE

Blood pressure is not significantly lowered during vigorous exercise. We must emphasize that during vigorous exercise such as five miles of jogging or 20 minutes of continuous aerobic exercise, the systolic blood pressure increases markedly in most individuals. In many, the rise in blood pressure is substantial and it is possible that damage can occur in arteries during vigorous exercise. For example, a 30-year-old with a normal systolic blood pressure of 120 mm Hg, on running one to two miles, will usually have an increase in blood pressure during the run to about 140 to 180; there is usually no increase in the diastolic blood pressure except in patients who have hypertension. Blood pressure rapidly falls on cessation of exercise and returns to the normal resting level within a few minutes. Individuals with mild hypertension who engage in a regular exercise program may obtain a slight reduction in their resting blood pressure, and this is believed to be due to a combination of factors, including weight loss and relaxation. Therefore, indirectly, regular exercises are important to assist with weight reduction, thereby lowering blood pressure in individuals with mild hypertension. If you have moderate or severe hypertension, do not depend on exercise; it will not reduce blood pressure and can cause an increase in existing high blood pressure during vigorous exercise. We cannot exclude the possibility that damage to arteries may be increased by vigorous exercise in some individuals.

EFFECTS ON THE BLOOD

Regular vigorous exercise increases high-density lipoprotein ("good") cholesterol from 1 to 10 percent. It is debatable whether this slight rise in HDL cholesterol decreases risk over a long period of time. Moderate exercise has a variable effect. The total blood cholesterol and low-density lipoprotein ("bad") cholesterol are not significantly reduced by exercise. Elevated triglycerides are reduced by exercise, but elevated triglycerides are not considered to be a risk factor for coronary heart disease.

Other effects of vigorous exercise include a variable effect on blood-clotting factors. A substance in the blood, factor VIII, is necessary for blood clotting and is absent in bleeders (hemophiliacs). Hemophiliacs who exercise get a mild and helpful increase in factor VIII. Vigorous exercise in healthy individuals increases factor VIII, as well as the number and stickiness of platelets. This is offset in healthy young individuals by a mild increase in factors that tend to dissolve blood clots. Individuals over age 50, or at any age if atherosclerosis of the artery is present, have an impaired ability to dissolve clots. Consequently, small clots (thrombi) may form on plaques of atheroma, thus increasing their size; and slowly, over five to 10 years, this may cause or promote existing coronary heart disease. Walking at a rate of four miles per hour, however, does not cause an increase in factor VIII or platelets, and the stickiness of platelets is slightly reduced. Therefore, "Walk and win! Miles for millions."

EXERCISE AND PREVENTION OF HEART TROUBLE

Millions of North Americans participate in regular exercise programs. This is a major achievement motivated by various advertisements and literature and the desire to feel fit as well as possibly to stay alive longer.

A few studies have suggested that cardiac death is more common in sedentary individuals than in the physically active. But further analysis of these studies revealed major defects in methodology and interpretation. Published studies on exercise and the risk of coronary heart disease lack standardization of the diagnosis of coronary heart disease, information on the effects of associated risk factors and reliable evaluation of recreational or occupational physical activity.

Studies include the following:

- To assess the role of physical exertion in relation to risk of fatal heart attack, the 1951-1972 work experience of 6,351 San Francisco longshoremen was studied. Among men age 35 to 54 there were 24 heart attack deaths in those engaged in heavy work, 37 deaths in men classified as doing moderate work and 28 deaths in those engaged in light work.

Thus, there was no difference in the death rates in men age 35 to 54. Among men age 65 to 74 there were 8 deaths in men engaged in heavy work six months prior to death, 9 deaths in those engaged in moderate work and 275 deaths in those engaged in light work six months before death. Each man who had a fatal heart attack was classified in the job category that he held six months before death. This study is controversial because of errors in methodology. Men 64 plus are usually engaged in light work activity and death is expected in this age group. We know that the 275 men over 64 who died were engaged in light work six months prior to death, but the study does not indicate what their activity level was during age 35 to 64.

- A study done in 1966 showed that London bus drivers had a slightly higher incidence of heart attacks than London bus conductors, but other risk factors confounded the analysis. For example, from the outset, the bus drivers were heavier, with a higher blood pressure and blood cholesterol than bus conductors and were, therefore, at higher risk. These risk factors were probably more important than job activity classification.

- In a seven-country collaborative study, moderately active Finns had a 2 1/2 times higher incidence of coronary heart disease than the least active and the most active Finns. Confounding factors in this study included a high incidence of elevated blood cholesterol, which may have modified the effects of increased physical activity.

- In a study of 17,000 male university alumni, 2,000 kilocalories (kcal) of exercise per week slightly reduced the risk of coronary heart disease. Vigorous sports, climbing stairs and walking to obtain a minimum of 500 kcal of exercise per week appeared to be necessary to obtain a reduced coronary artery disease risk.

- An Australian group studied 370 men who took part in a twice-weekly exercise program with one hour of calisthenics, volleyball and running so as to improve physical fitness by 17 percent. The program was continued for five years, and even though the men felt physically fit, there was no reduction in blood cholesterol, weight, or blood pressure.

- Morris et al. analyzed the exercise habits of 18,000 sedentary male office workers. Those with vigorous leisure time activity had about a 50 percent reduction in heart attacks. The 18,000 men were asked on a Monday morning to complete a record indicating their level of physical activity on the preceding Friday and Saturday. In this study, vigorous exercise included (a) sports and recreation, i.e., singles tennis, swimming, jogging, running, walking at a rate of four miles per hour and cycling fast uphill; and (b) very heavy work. At the end of 8 1/2 years, there were 24 (1.1 percent) fatal and 42 (2 percent) nonfatal heart attacks in the vigorous-exercise group of 2,200 men, but 411 (2.4 percent) fatal and 570 (3.4 percent) nonfatal heart attacks in the nonvigorous-exercise group of 16,800 men. Thus there was about a 50 percent reduction in heart attacks attributed to the good effects of vigorous exercise. These results are statistically significant. However, selection of individuals may have created a bias and the study can be criticized.

- Marathon running does not offer any guarantees, and it is not believed to be as protective as some enthusiasts would have us believe. In four of seven marathoners who had completed a total of 64 marathons and died, autopsy showed severe atherosclerosis of their coronary arteries. The bad news is that severe coronary atherosclerosis is the commonest cause of death, even among marathoners.

- A study reported in the *New England Journal of Medicine*, June 1994, gives support to the notion that lower levels of physical activity appear to increase the risk of coronary heart disease. Very high levels of physical activity may confer some protection.

It is worth noting that in Finland there is a high occupational level of physical exertion, yet coronary heart disease mortality is very high.

The public must understand that exercise has important benefits, *but it cannot be expected to halt the progression or complications of coronary heart disease, and attention to other risk factors is necessary* .

RISKS OF EXERCISE

The relationship between vigorous exercise and the risk of a fatal or nonfatal heart attack has long been the subject of controversy. A study reported in the *New England Journal of Medicine*, October 1984, showed that vigorous exercise can precipitate sudden cardiac death in healthy individuals. The risk of sudden death is higher in men with low levels of habitual activity who engage in unusual vigorous exercise. Even in men who were accustomed to vigorous activity, however, the risk of sudden cardiac death was moderately increased during high-intensity exercise. This study did create a stir.

We must emphasize that the authors only analyzed nine deaths. It would be foolhardy to make any generalizations from such a study. The study was done in King County, Washington, an area containing 1.25 million people. Only nine cardiac arrests during vigorous exercise occurred in 14 months — five in men with low levels of habitual activity and four in men with high levels of activity. This study should not influence the medical profession or public except to emphasize that jogging is relatively safe and cardiac arrest is very rare. However, sedentary individuals should not rush out and do vigorous exercises without engaging in levels of gradual activity. In addition, in Rhode Island during a six-year period, only one jogging death occurred per year for every 6,720 joggers. This is a very low death rate but is higher than expected. Despite our defense of jogging for those who love it, we must emphasize that all studies show a much higher incidence of heart attacks during exercise than would be expected by chance. Heart attack is the commonest cause of death during exercise.

The death of exercise enthusiast James Fixx is a good example of nonprotection by exercise. In his early 30s he recognized that he was at high risk since his family history was strong for heart attacks before age 50. A daily run of five to 10 miles for more than 15 years did not protect him from the silent killer.

Note that during jogging and running, the systolic blood pressure may be slightly or moderately increased. The combined increase in blood pressure and high-velocity blood flow may over a period of years increase atherosclerosis.

Strenuous exercise can precipitate death in individuals who have a very rare heart muscle problem called obstructive cardiomyopathy. The division (septum) between the right and left ventricle becomes extremely thick for reasons unknown and obstructs the blood flow from the left ventricle into the aorta. This condition explains the rare sudden death that occurs in some athletes under the age of 30. This obstructive heart muscle problem is fortunately very rare and is easy to exclude by a doctor listening with a stethoscope and with added tests such as an ECG and an echocardiogram.

All patients with known heart disease or with symptoms that suggest heart disease — pain or discomfort in the chest, throat, jaw or arms during activity; shortness of breath; palpitations (fast, pounding heartbeats or skipped heartbeats) — should have an assessment by a doctor and a stress test before engaging in moderate or vigorous exercise. Patients with previous heart failure or marked heart enlargement should engage only in moderate exercise such as walking or its equivalent. Exercise is well known to precipitate heart failure in such individuals, and therefore further advice from your doctor is necessary if you want to do exercise other than the equivalent of walking one mile.

Injuries During Jogging

The up and down motion of jogging causes tendon, muscle, and joint injuries. In one survey, about 1,800 injuries occurred in 1,650 amateur runners. Injuries included: 1) Achilles' tendinitis: the heel and the tendon become painful; 2) shin splints: the muscles at the front of the leg (frontal compartment syndrome) become painful and swollen; 3) painful knees: inflammation of the fluid-filled sac (bursitis), strain on ligaments, or painful knee caps (chondromalacia patellae); 4) painful feet: inflammation of the sole of the foot, plantar fasciitis and trauma to the bones of the foot; and 5) exacerbation of arthritis of the hips, knees and ankles. Patients with arthritis must not jog. Women are more susceptible to knee injuries or stress fractures in the pelvis, and in some, osteoporosis (loss of bone) may develop.

If you must jog, purchase good running shoes, exercise the ankle joint and warm up properly to prevent injuries. Despite such precautions, injuries are very common among joggers.

How to Start an Exercise Program

If you are under 35, do not have arthritis or moderate or severe hypertension and feel in good health, you can engage in all activities, including vigorous exercise, as frequently as you desire. Regardless of age, it is wise to do five to 10 minutes of warm-up exercises before going on to vigorous exercises. Warm-up exercises prevent the pulse and blood pressure from increasing abruptly, thereby putting sudden strain on the heart. You should engage for one to two weeks in moderate exercise such as walking one to two miles or jogging one mile daily before considering vigorous aerobic exercise such as running two to five miles three or four times weekly. If you are under 35, there is very little reason to check the pulse rate. If you feel your heart pounding away very rapidly, then slow your pace. For those engaged in competitive sports: we are in agreement with other experts, that running is perhaps the best exercise for those who require the stamina to do the utmost. The swimmer, boxer or cyclist should jog to develop stamina and strengthen other muscles. Similarly, the runner should engage in other exercises, especially swimming and cycling.

For individuals over age 35 in good health, the following advice is given:

- Walking two miles in a half hour, swimming and cycling are excellent exercises. They are efficient and safe, as well as economical. Walking four miles in an hour and climbing six flights of stairs daily can produce cardiovascular conditioning. You do not require special equipment and you do not have to travel to a gym or ski slope or racquet club. Walking two miles quickly burns up as many calories as jogging one mile. Jogging exercises the legs but not the important quadriceps muscles at the front of the thighs. Walking up three to six flights of stairs daily or cycling will strengthen the quadriceps; strong quadriceps strengthen and stabilize the knees.
- If you are physically inactive at work and at home for more than six months, you should start very slowly. Start with daily or alternate-day 10-minute stretching exercises, moving all the joints and the muscles of the upper and lower limbs as well as the trunk. Follow with 20 minutes of brisk walking (a little more than a mile), and then cycle for five to 10 minutes. A stationary bicycle or treadmill is a good investment.

After about four weeks of this mild exercise, increase the walk to 30 minutes and cycle for 10 to 15 minutes. After one month of this routine, if you feel well with no abnormal symptoms such as chest, throat or arm discomfort, very fast heartbeats or shortness of breath, you can freely engage in your favorite racquet sport. Swimming is well known to be an excellent conditioner as well as pleasurable exercise. If you wish to move to vigorous exercise, you should have a medical checkup. It is a pity that many individuals commence regular jogging or other exercise at 28 and stop at 38. For some it is a pleasure and for others an obsession that imposes stress. Those who love jogging should obviously continue, especially through the vulnerable years — ages 35 to 55.

Heart Rate Maximum and Training Range

Learn to take your heart rate and determine your maximal and submaximal heart rate. During your medical checkup, your doctor will show you how to feel the pulse at the wrist (radial artery) or the carotid artery in the neck. Count the pulse beat for 10 seconds and multiply the number by six to get the heart rate per minute.

The heart rate increases to high levels with vigorous exercise, and these upper limits have been established by doctors engaged in exercise conditioning programs.

Several charts have been designed by experts and used in different countries. At age 20 the highest heart rate that the normal heart can achieve is between 200 and 220 beats per minute, and this is called the maximum attainable heart rate (Table 2). To be safe, doctors advise that you should not exceed 85 percent of this maximal value, that is, about 170 per minute if you are young and healthy. During the first few weeks of training, keep the heart rate at about 70 percent maximum, that is, about 140 beats per minute, and increase the exercise to 85 percent if you are under age 30. If you are in good health, it is safe to exercise so that your heart rate reaches 70 to 85 percent of your maximal and to keep it at this rate for about 20 minutes. After six to eight weeks of strenuous exercise, you should achieve physical and cardiopulmonary conditioning. At age 40 your maximum heart rate should be approximately 220 minus 40, or 180, and your training range — your "target zone" — from 125 to 150; i.e., your pulse counted for 10 seconds should be a minimum of 20 and a maximum of 25 beats. We must emphasize that you do not necessarily need to reach and maintain the target zone, as some have claimed, to obtain conditioning — the training effect.

TABLE 2 Age-Related Maximum Attainable Heart Rates and Training Range										
Age	20	25	30	35	40	45	50	55	60	65
Maximum Heart Rate (220 - age)	200	195	190	185	180	175	170	165	160	155
85% Training Zone	170	165	161	157	153	148	144	140	136	131
70%	140	136	133	130	126	122	119	115	112	108

Maximum rates and training ranges are given in Table 2. Individuals over age 40 who have not engaged in strenuous exercise in the last two years or who have a family history of heart attacks before age 50, blood cholesterol greater than 220 mg or mild hypertension, are advised to have a stress test before starting vigorous exercise.

EXERCISE STRESS TEST

A stress test involves walking on the treadmill or cycling while your ECG is being continuously recorded. The ECG terminals are taped onto your chest. Walking on the treadmill is easier if you wear running shoes or other comfortable flat shoes. The treadmill speed and its inclination are programmed to increase every three minutes so that you walk faster up a grade and are jogging by the 10th minute. Healthy individuals are exercised to 90 percent of their maximal heart rate. The test is discontinued if chest or leg pain, fatigue or shortness of breath develops or if the electrocardiogram shows insufficient oxygen to the heart muscle. The blood pressure is taken every three minutes, and the systolic blood pressure usually rises by 20 to 40 mm Hg. A 40-year-old who is physically fit with good cardiopulmonary condition can usually exercise for 10 to 12 minutes, reaching a heart rate of 160 to 170 beats per minute, without having undue shortness of breath. The test is completed by a few minutes of slow walking to cool down before the treadmill is turned off.

A well-conditioned 35-year-old athlete's heart rate may increase only to 140 per minute during 12 minutes of such exercise; on resting, the heart rate should fall quickly to under 100 per minute within one to four minutes. The same cool-down period should apply in your exercise regime at home. When you have completed your vigorous exercise, always cool down for two to five minutes by walking around, doing some stretching, or going up and down stairs a few times.

Exercise prescriptions for patients who have heart disease, especially coronary heart disease, are discussed under Heart Attacks and Rehabilitation.

CONCLUSION

We strongly recommend regular, moderate exercise for healthy individuals and those with coronary or mild valvular heart disease. Fitness makes one feel like living and confers a sense of well-being. If you are relatively fit, you can enjoy your favorite sport with better breathing capabilities and without feeling your heart pounding. If you are fit, you are not likely to be overweight, your clothes fit you better and you feel and look better. We strongly recommend regular moderate exercise to achieve a state of "relative fitness."

We recommend vigorous exercise to those who are healthy and already fit. A fit heart idles at a slower speed. A heart that beats slower allows better filling of normal or partially obstructed coronary arteries. There is no scientific proof or adequate evidence, however, to suggest that vigorous exercise will make you live longer. If you are over age 40, mainly sedentary, and engage in occasional mild exercise, do not start vigorous exercise without having a medical check or stress test. Start with walking one to two miles daily, slowly adding cycling, swimming or similar exercise. Avoid vigorous exercise until you have done more than three months of daily moderate exercise.

Vigorous exercise in previously inactive individuals over age 35 carries a high risk of fatal or nonfatal heart attacks or sudden death. Therefore, do not rush to get superfit. Get fit slowly over three to six months, remembering that fitness is a relative term — fit to do what?

In addition, we emphasize that simple exercises — walking two miles in a half hour or when possible four miles in an hour, climbing stairs or peddling a stationary bicycle for 15 minutes — are excellent safe exercises. Walking is always helpful and "never" causes a heart attack. It does not increase blood pressure; it improves circulation in the legs and may have a favorable influence on blood clotting. Therefore, if you walk, you may win the *race*!

FAINTING/SYNCOPE

A simple faint is a common occurrence: A faint and other forms of loss of consciousness lasting a few seconds caused by lack of blood to the brain is medically termed syncope. Recovery is rapid if the head is kept lower than the legs so that blood can be delivered more efficiently to the brain. Placing the individual flat on the ground with the legs elevated is the quickest method of getting blood to the brain, and the person rapidly regains consciousness.

A faint is heralded by a feeling of weakness, lightheadedness and sometimes nausea. These symptoms may be present for a few seconds or for a couple of minutes prior to the individual falling to the ground. Often there is sufficient warning to allow the individual to get to a sitting position and to put the head between the knees. Fainting usually occurs in certain settings: the individual may have been standing for too long; blood pools in the legs, less blood reaches the brain and weakness with transient loss of consciousness may occur.

Some individuals have a propensity to fainting spells. Fainting may be precipitated by drugs that lower blood pressure excessively. Mitral valve prolapse, blood loss, severe vomiting and diarrhea causing dehydration and high fevers may precipitate attacks. Syncope is not usually associated with abnormal movements of the limbs; such seizure activity may be accompanied by incontinence or tongue biting, which is not observed with a faint.

Heart conditions may cause syncope or a faint-like feeling. Occasionally this is caused by an abnormally slow heart rate of less than 40 beats per minute. This form of disturbance in the electrical conduction of the heart may require the implantation of a pacemaker (see Pacemakers). Individuals who experience loss of consciousness for a period of seconds or minutes without residual weakness in the limbs and without the precipitating factors mentioned above should consult a physician to check for the possibility of abnormal heart rhythms.

FISH/FISH OILS

The low mortality from coronary heart disease in Greenland Inuit is attributed to their intake of more than 350 g per day of whale and seal meat. In Japan, the incidence of coronary heart disease is much lower in areas where fish consumption is high, but the alpha-linolenic acid in soybeans and other products may be responsible for the low mortality from heart disease.

Fatty fish contains omega n-3 fatty acids represented mainly by eicosapentaenoic and docosahexaenoic acids. These agents have an aspirin-like effect that prevents blood platelets from clumping together; this action prevents clot formation. They also have other beneficial effects on the walls of the arteries.

Nonetheless, studies of large populations in Norway and Japanese men in the Honolulu Heart Program showed no beneficial effect of fish intake on cardiovascular disease. In contrast, however, a study in 872 men followed from 1960 to 1980 showed a 40 percent reduction in the risk of death from coronary heart disease in those who ate an average of 70 grams of fish a week compared with those who did not eat fish. The Western Electric Study of 1,931 men followed for 25 years showed some reduction in coronary heart disease mortality in men eating approximately 60 g of fish per week compared with those who ate no fish. These nonrandomized studies have many limitations, however, and may not answer questions adequately.

In a small, randomized trial of diet in 2,033 men who had had a previous heart attack, it was found that consuming two servings of 200 to 400 g of fatty fish per week for two years caused a significant reduction in mortality and nonfatal heart attacks. Because this clinical trial and other surveys show a positive trend for protection from heart attacks, we conclude that it is advisable for individuals over age 25 to eat two servings of 175 g (6 oz) of fatty fish weekly. Individuals with a family history of heart attacks before age 60 and those who have had a heart attack should use this simple nondrug protective regimen. Fatty fish includes salmon, tuna, mackerel, cod and herring. A large study reported in the *New England Journal of Medicine,* April 1995, indicates that any beneficial effect is obtained with one or two servings of fish per week and that more is not better.

GARLIC/ONIONS

There is some experimental data suggesting that 60 milligrams of fried or boiled onions can normalize the increase in lipid content and clotting properties of the blood induced by a fatty meal. Garlic appears to have a similar favorable effect. Sound scientific evidence is lacking. Other plant materials are being investigated.

HEART ATTACKS

CAUSES

The cause of a heart attack in the majority of cases is a blockage of a coronary artery by a blood clot. The clot usually occurs on the surface of a partially obstructing plaque of atheroma (see Figs. 1 and 3) The surface of a plaque ruptures and the plaque contains substances that increase the clotting of blood. A clot therefore forms on the surface of the rupture and also inside the plaque.

In the majority of patients who have a heart attack, no precipitating factor can be identified. The individual may wonder, why today? What did I do wrong? Only occasionally is there some circumstantial evidence that may be related, for example, excessive unaccustomed exertion or severe stress. A large fatty meal, bed rest for several months and overwork without undue distress do not appear to be precipitating factors. No one knows when a plaque of atheroma will rupture and cause a clot. If the blood is thicker and has a greater tendency to clot than normal, the individual is obviously at greater risk of having a heart attack. Substances that cause rapid and intense clotting are released when the plaque ruptures; these substances are exposed to the flowing blood and a clot quickly forms, thus blocking the artery.

Possibly, new drugs could be produced to inhibit the clotting substances in the plaque. We offer this hypothesis with the hope that a pharmaceutical firm or scientist will explore the possibility and produce a product that can prevent a fatal or nonfatal heart attack. The simple drug aspirin certainly helps to prevent some heart attacks and save lives but does not nullify the clotting properties of the ruptured plaque contents.

When a heart attack begins, the individual is suddenly stricken by pain in the center of the chest. The pain is often unbearable and may be a pressure-like discomfort accompanied by difficult breathing, profuse sweating and a strange frightened feeling. The cause of a heart attack in the majority of cases is a blockage of a coronary artery that feeds the heart muscle with blood containing oxygen, glucose, sodium, potassium, calcium and other nutrients. In more than 90 percent of patients, the blockage has been shown conclusively to be due to a blood clot. The blood clot is often present on the surface of a partially obstructing plaque of atheroma (atherosclerosis) that shows fissuring (rupture or ulceration). The blocked artery cuts off blood to a segment of heart muscle (myocardium), the cells of which die because they are deprived of the nutrients in the blood. This death of heart muscle cells is termed a myocardial infarction (see Fig. 1). After a few months this area of dead muscle forms a well-healed scar. The size of the myocardial infarction depends on the coronary artery affected, i.e., a main vessel or a branch artery, and what part of the heart muscle it supplies. A heart attack is synonymous with the term "myocardial infarction" and, for practical purposes, with "coronary thrombosis." If the anterior part of the heart is involved, this is more serious than involvement of the back (inferior) part of the heart. Inferior infarction has a very good prognosis.

In the majority of individuals, the cause of a heart attack is a clot (thrombosis) in one of the coronary arteries; the clot can be dissolved by special drugs that we will discuss later in this section. For this treatment to be most effective, it should be given within four hours from the onset of the symptoms of a heart attack, that is, four hours from the onset of chest pain, which is the most common symptom. Beyond six hours, the chance of success with this treatment is remote, since the heart muscle cells become irreversibly damaged and die between two and five hours after the blood supply has been cut off. Many patients are given treatment from six to 12 hours after the onset of their symptoms with the hope of saving a few lives. The number of lives saved by treating 1,000 patients with thrombolytic therapy given at less than one, three, six and 12 hours from the onset of symptoms are 65, 27, 25 and eight, respectively. Widespread advice to the population at risk is crucial. Less than 15 percent of heart attack victims presently receive therapy within four hours of the onset of symptoms. Only about 30 percent of patients receive treatment within six hours.

We strongly advise you to learn the symptoms and signs of a heart attack (see Signs and Symptoms). If you think you or someone else is experiencing a heart attack, you should go immediately to the nearest emergency room of a hospital. All hospitals have the facilities to give drugs that dissolve clots in the coronary arteries. This life-saving treatment is usually given within minutes of your arrival. *If you need to wait more than 20 minutes* to receive the drug, your spouse or person accompanying you to the hospital should raise hell! The wait in most hospitals exceeds 40 minutes. A wait of more than 20 minutes is *inexcusable.*

SIGNS AND SYMPTOMS

The symptoms of a heart attack are often typical and easy to recognize. In some patients, however, symptoms can be so varied that both the patient and the doctor can be misled. People have unique feelings and sensations and use different words to describe similar symptoms. Heart attacks vary a great deal in their severity, and patients are not all alike. Thus, the characteristics of pain and the accompanying symptoms can be very different from one individual to another.

People experiencing a heart attack often have difficulty describing the type of pain or peculiar discomfort or distress. Some words used by various patients to describe the discomfort are listed so that you can learn to recognize the peculiar sensation:

- *Crushing or compressing pain or a heaviness over the chest.* The pain is most often described as "a crushing pain across my chest." Or the patient states that it feels like a very heavy weight or bar is resting on the center of the chest, especially over the breastbone (sternum), or, "It feels as if someone is crushing or walking on my chest."
- *Viselike tightness, squeezing, constricting.* It feels as if the chest is in a vise or as if a tight metal band is being pulled around the chest. The constricting feeling is often described as a tightness. The patient tries to describe the tightness by clenching a fist.
- *A disagreeable choking, strangling, sickening feeling in the center and across the chest.* This type of sensation can occur

in patients with anxiety and may not be due to a heart attack. This strangling sensation is, however, very important because it resembles the discomfort in patients with angina pectoris. Patients with angina can develop chest discomfort mainly on exertion due to a lack of blood supply to the heart muscle. If the strangling sensation comes on at rest and lasts for more than 30 minutes and especially if it is accompanied by the associated symptoms of a heart attack, you should seek attention.

- *Burning-like indigestion.* A burning discomfort or pain in the center of the chest, especially when accompanied by sweating or sensations listed under associated symptoms, must be taken seriously as it can be caused by a heart attack. Pain originating from the stomach is often burning in quality, but the associated symptoms differentiate heart from stomach pain. For example, heart pain is very often associated with profuse sweating, whereas stomach pain rarely ever causes sweating.

- *Tearing, gripping pain,* as if the chest were being pulled apart from the breastbone.

- *Fullness in the chest,* as if it wanted to explode, may be a symptom of a heart attack, but it can be due to pain originating from the stomach or gullet (esophagus), for example, gas pains, or to reflux esophagitis.

- *Just a discomfort.* The patient may not perceive the sensation as pain but as a mild to moderate discomfort. Such a discomfort is a common feature and must not be ignored, especially if associated signs and symptoms are present.

- *Tingling, numbness, or heaviness* over the left or right arm may occur at the same time as the pain in the chest but is rarely the only manifestation of a heart attack. However, there are many causes of such symptoms in the arms, especially pain from the nerves supplying the arms, muscular pain or a small stroke, in which case, the hand and the arm will be very weak. A heart attack does not cause the arm or hand to become severely weak and it never causes paralysis.

- *A pointed, sharp, stabbing, sticking, knifelike pain* is seldom a manifestation of a heart attack. Such chest pain is often produced by other sources, such as the chest wall or the lungs, as in pleurisy and gas pains.

- *Dizziness and/or severe weakness* commonly occurs along with the chest pain of a heart attack, but is rarely the only symptom.

- *Nausea without vomiting or diarrhea*, if associated with pain in the chest or discomfort or shortness of breath, weakness or dizziness, can be a symptom of a heart attack and rarely occurs without chest pain. In such a situation, associated shortness of breath points to a disturbance of the heart, rather than the stomach.
- *Aching pain under the breastbone or arm* is occasionally described by patients.

The Location of the Pain

In the majority of individuals, the pain of a heart attack is in the center of the chest under the breastbone (retrosternal). The pain is more often located under the lower two-thirds of the breastbone (see Fig. 5). Note that the heart projects to the left side of the breastbone and pain under or outside of the nipple line rarely comes from a heart attack.

The next most common area is the upper half of the breastbone and the pit of the stomach. Heart pain occurs mainly in the center of the chest, and doctors often use the term "central retrosternal chest pain" as being typical of a heart attack. Finally, pain from all three areas can move (radiate) up or down to involve the entire chest, neck, throat and lower jaw (not higher than the upper jaw) and commonly extends to the arms, forearms and hands. Both arms may feel painful, heavy, numb or tingly. Left arm discomfort is more common than right, and as shown in Figure 5 area 2, the inner aspect (ulnar side of the arm) is the commonest site of arm pain. Most of the arm or a small part such as the wrist may be the site of pain or discomfort without involvement of the chest. However, arm, jaw or throat pain is usually acompanied by pain in the chest. If pain is present only in the upper limb, the accompanying symptoms and signs of a heart attack then become very important in making the diagnosis. For example, if there is associated shortness of breath, nausea and sudden generalized weakness, the arm pain can be the manifestation of a heart attack.

Pain below the level of the belly button (umbilicus) is not from the heart. In addition, the pain of a heart attack very rarely goes through to the back. If it does, it is usually the zone between the left shoulder blade and the spine. Pain only in the area on both sides of a vertical line drawn through the nipple is most unlikely

to be due to a heart attack (see Fig. 5). Centrally located breastbone pain can radiate across the entire chest, that is, to the left
and occasionally to the right of the nipple line and upward to the
neck and jaw. Thus, while in some cases, the size of the area may
be that of one to three clenched fists or the entire span of the
palm and outstretched fingers, pain can involve the entire front of
the chest.

The Severity and Duration of the Pain

The pain of a heart attack varies in intensity. In about 50 percent
of patients, it is described as severe pain. In about 10 percent of
patients, it is very severe and unbearable. In about 20 percent
of patients, the pain is a moderate pain that is not in itself distressing and may well be a mild discomfort not reaching the level
of pain. In such patients, the associated symptoms are important,
especially the feeling of anguish or fear of impending doom,
which is common in patients who are having a heart attack. In
about 10 percent of cases, there is profound weakness, sweating,
dizziness, nausea or palpitations. In the remaining 10 percent of
cases, particularly in diabetics and in the elderly, no symptoms
occur and a heart attack is discovered only on subsequent routine
electrocardiographic or autopsy examinations.

The pain of heart attack usually lasts more than 30 minutes and
frequently one to four hours. A pain that lasts less than one
minute and returns each time only to last a couple of minutes is
usually not due to a heart attack, especially if there are no other
associated symptoms. Pain lasting less than 10 seconds, even
when recurrent, is not due to a heart attack. The pain of angina
usually lasts from one to five minutes and its maximum is 15 minutes. If the pain is similar to the accustomed anginal pain but now
lasts more than 20 minutes, especially if you are at rest, you must
seriously consider the possibility of a heart attack and have the
situation assessed in a hospital emergency room. Diabetics
and people over age 75 may have little or no pain during a heart
attack. The elderly may get weakness or shortness of breath
without chest pain.

The pain of a heart attack can come on gradually over a half to
one hour with increasing intensity that may remain steady for a
few hours. It is usually a steady pain, not an on-and-off pain such
as occurs with crampy stomach problems or abdominal pain that

is usually described as colic (colicky or spasmodic pain). After one to four hours, the pain of a heart attack may suddenly disappear never to return and the individual may feel fairly well. The patient may no longer be disturbed and can make the mistake of not going to an emergency room or of leaving the hospital. Pain ceases as the heart muscle cells die when they are deprived of blood. *Dead muscle cells produce no pain.* On rare occasions, pain may persist for six to 12 hours in three or four bouts each lasting a few hours, and between times, a dull pressure, tightness, heaviness or ache remains somewhere in the center of the chest or areas described above.

Warning Attacks

About 20 to 30 percent of patients who have a heart attack experience a "warning" some time during the two weeks prior to the attack. Patients who have chest pain (angina) suddenly notice a change in the duration and frequency of the pain. Instead of lasting one to five minutes, the pain may last five to 20 minutes and is brought on with less activity and may even occur at rest. This usually indicates that the angina is progressing or unstable. If the pain lasts longer than 30 minutes and is not relieved by two nitroglycerin tablets, it is likely due to a heart attack. If the pain lasts from 15 to 30 minutes, it is likely due to unstable angina that can lead to a heart attack over the next few months. In such a situation, you can prevent a heart attack if you get proper attention.

In patients who are not known to have angina, pain may suddenly come on for the first time during a bout of unaccustomed exertion such as shoveling snow, pushing a car, hauling a boat or running. Chest pain or discomfort may last only two to 10 minutes and may be ignored only to return in full force within a few days. If pain occurs for only a few minutes, take special note if the pain is relieved within one to two minutes after stopping the precipitating activity. About 25 percent of such patients are likely to have a heart attack within the next month, which may be prevented by the combination of a beta-blocking drug and one aspirin daily. In addition, the electrocardiogram is usually normal in such patients when pain is absent. Thus, they are often sent away from the emergency room. This must not deter you from seeking appropriate expert medical care.

Associated Symptoms

As discussed above, pain or discomfort of a heart attack is nearly always accompanied by one or more symptoms that may help you or the doctor clarify the diagnosis. Therefore, identifying these associated symptoms is of vital importance.

1. *Sweating* is often profuse for at least a few minutes. In particular, the forehead is usually covered with a cold sweat. Indigestion or stomach pains that can be confused with a heart attack do not usually cause profuse sweating. It is well known that sweating occurs during a fever as the temperature rises above 100°F (38°C). A heart attack, however, does not cause a rise in body temperature until about the second day. Therefore, if you have sudden pain and definite fever, it is most unlikely to be due to a heart attack.

2. *Difficulty breathing* is very common and may last for a few minutes. Persistence of shortness of breath for more than 10 minutes suggests that blood and fluid are accumulating in the lungs due to heart failure and requires prompt attention. Shortness of breath must be distinguished from sighing respirations, which involve taking one or two deep breaths and completely exhaling. Sighing is a common occurrence in individuals who are under stress and can be due to tiredness, exhaustion or anxiety. Difficulty breathing can mean several things: You cannot take a deep breath because your chest hurts — for example, if a rib is fractured or there is an infection on the outer surface of the lung membrane (pleurisy). Moving the chest wall produces lung pain; therefore, a deep breath cannot be taken because it causes pain and the individual is forced to take shallow breaths. Shortness of breath is a different sensation, and it means that you feel out of breath and are forced to gasp and struggle for breath, breathing rapidly and shallowly. The feeling is similar to that of running up four or five flights of stairs. Afterward, you are out of breath and have to breathe harder and quicker. During heart failure the lungs have extra water and blood and become "stiff," making a very deep breath impossible; therefore, breathing tends to be a little shallow. When shortness of breath is due to heart trouble, it is made worse by lying flat and can improve a little if the individual sits up and dangles the legs. Some nervous and anxious individuals

hyperventilate, and this must be differentiated from true shortness of breath.

To re-emphasize, the pain of a heart attack is not increased by taking a very deep breath, coughing or sneezing.

3. *A feeling of impending doom* is experienced by virtually all patients who are having a heart attack. This fear and anxiety can provoke the secretion of adrenaline and noradrenaline, which increases heart damage and may disturb the heart rhythm. The increase in adrenaline causes irritability of the dying heart muscle and triggers the production of extra beats and occasionally may result in ventricular fibrillation, during which the heart muscle does not contract but quivers. It is imperative that pain, fear and anxiety be quickly relieved with adequate pain-relieving drugs such as morphine, oxygen and with reassurance by a doctor. You will reassure yourself if you quickly reach a hospital where adequate facilities exist to relieve pain and combat your heart attack.

One of our patients, a male age 48, had several typical symptoms during his heart attack: he suddenly experienced a disagreeable sensation in the chest, which increased to a heavy crushing sensation over and beneath the lower part of the breastbone. During the next 10 to 15 minutes, the pain felt like a heavy bar across the chest and within a few minutes spread to his left arm, which felt as heavy as lead. He was not known to have angina and therefore had no nitroglycerin available. He was overcome by a strange fear with a feeling that life was going to be extinguished. At this point, his pain had lasted about 40 minutes, and was moderately severe but could not be described as unbearable. He was sweating profusely and upon further questioning, he admitted that it was his fear that prompted him to call the ambulance. It is true that many people are afraid of a heart attack and may develop anxiety. Many individuals with pain in different parts of the body may become a little anxious, but few feel as if they are strangling, and this sensation seems to produce great fear and anxiety.

4. *Severe and sudden weakness* may be associated with chest discomfort in about one-third of patients with a heart attack. The heart muscle is damaged and cannot pump with maximum force. Less blood is ejected from the heart at each beat; therefore, blood pressure falls and less blood reaches the brain. Thus the patient may feel weak and feel like fainting.

Transient loss of consciousness for a couple of minutes can occur but is uncommon. The blood pressure soon becomes restored to near normal because of the body's compensatory responses, and weakness improves. In a few patients with a severe heart attack, the blood pressure remains very low and the weakness is profound (cardiogenic shock).

5. *Dizziness or light-headedness* may occur in some patients owing to a drop in blood pressure. Ringing in the ears (tinnitus) or severe rotational dizziness (vertigo) are not usually features of a heart attack.

6. *Nausea and occasionally vomiting* accompany the pain in a significant number of patients. Severe pain from any cause may precipitate vomiting, and pain relievers such as morphine usually increase nausea and vomiting. However, unaccustomed sudden nausea may occur instead of pain or chest discomfort. Thus, distressing nausea with sweating and shortness of breath should be considered due to a heart disturbance until proven otherwise.

7. *Restlessness* as the patient tries to find a comfortable position. However, the pain or discomfort of a heart attack is not relieved by any particular position. The pain is not made better or worse by sitting, standing, lying or rolling from side to side.

8. *Shortness of breath* if the heart muscle is very weak and heart failure occurs during the heart attack. The individual may be gasping. In such cases, some relief is obtained when the patient is propped up in bed.

9. *A cough* may suddenly develop with the production of frothy pink or blood-stained sputum.

10. *A sharp drop in blood pressure* may occur, signaled by confusion and loss of consciousness, if the heart attack is very severe, because of the lack of oxygen to the brain. Loss of consciousness is rare and a loss for more than two minutes is not a feature of heart attacks. When the heart muscle is suddenly weakened by a heart attack, the blood pressure may fall 10 to 40 mm of Hg and the pulse may become rapid. Thus in about half of patients with heart attacks, the systolic blood pressure may fall from an average of 125 mm to less than 105 mm. However, during the next few hours, if the heart attack is not a very large one, the body's compensatory responses may be sufficient to increase the blood pressure to the normal systolic range for the individual. The

fall in blood pressure caused by a heart attack often reduces the blood pressure of a hypertensive patient to normal so that medications for high blood pressure may not be required for several months and in some cases forever.

Patients with known coronary heart disease and perhaps all males over 40 and females over 50 would be wise to invest in a blood pressure instrument (sphygmomanometer). A doctor can teach you how to measure blood pressure and then you, your spouse or a friend can take it every six months so that you know your average blood pressure reading (see Hypertension and Measurement of Blood Pressure). Thus, if you are worried about chest discomfort or indigestion that is not relieved by an antacid and your systolic blood pressure falls more than 30 mm below the average baseline, this should prompt a visit to an emergency room. If you are in doubt because the discomfort seems to be in the stomach, an associated fall in blood pressure may warn you and save your life. On the other hand, since not all patients have a fall in blood pressure and the rare patient may have a mild increase in blood pressure because of pain and nervous reflexes, do not wait for a fall in blood pressure if chest pain with other associated symptoms is present; go to the emergency room.

11. *A change in heart rate accompanied by chest discomfort* may indicate that a heart attack is under way. We feel it is important for everyone over the age of 35 to learn how to determine the heart rate by feeling the pulse at the wrist. Then if you experience chest discomfort, the pulse decreases by 20 or increases by 20 when you are at rest, this is likely to be a warning of a heart attack. For example, if your resting pulse rate is usually in the range of 70 to 80 beats per minute and you suddenly find it at 50 to 60 beats per minute while having chest discomfort, the disturbance likely originates from the heart, especially if you are not on medication such as beta-blockers, which slow the pulse rate. A reduction in heart rate of 10 or less is too small to be diagnostic.

If the back of the heart muscle is affected during the attack (inferior heart attack), the pulse usually slows. If the front part of the heart muscle is affected (anterior heart attack), the pulse usually increases by 20 to 40 beats per minute and can reach 100 to 120 beats per minute at rest.

We would strongly suggest that if you have coronary heart disease or if you are over 45, your home should be equipped with a blood pressure instrument, nitroglycerin and plain aspirin. These are as essential as having a smoke detector or a fire extinguisher in the home. It is far more important to learn the symptoms and signs of a heart attack and the procedure for measuring your blood pressure and taking your pulse than it is to learn about cardiopulmonary resuscitation (CPR).

MIMICS

Several conditions cause symptoms that can mimic heart attacks. These are the most common:

- Indigestion and reflux esophagitis, hiatus hernia and esophageal spasm
- Lung infections: pleurisy and pneumonia
- Pericarditis
- Chest wall pain originating from the muscles, ribs, intercostal nerves or costochondral joints, or due to a common condition, costochondritis
- Arm pain, tingling and numbness in the left or right upper limb, not related to exertion such as a brisk walk

Rest assured that about half of all patients admitted to the hospital because of chest pain are not having a heart attack. These patients usually have an unstable form of angina pectoris, chest wall pain, stomach problems (in particular, reflux esophagitis with esophageal spasm), gallstones and very rarely pericarditis. Occasionally no cause can be found.

Indigestion and Stomach Problems

Those of you who have indigestion can distinguish it from the symptoms or discomfort caused by a heart attack. Pain of a heart attack can be present in the pit of the stomach (upper epigastrium) and the lower sternal area and may even be burning in type. Burning pain is more common with stomach and esophageal pain and is relieved by antacids, but the burning caused by a heart attack is not relieved by antacids. Associated profuse sweating or shortness of breath points to a heart attack rather than stomach or esophageal pain. Pain from ulcers in the stomach does not cause sweating, is related to meals and is often relieved by antacids.

Reflux Esophagitis and Hiatus Hernia

A sphincter, called the cardiac sphincter, is present at the junction of the esophagus and stomach (see Fig. 5). This sphincter closes tightly when an individual is at rest, but relaxes and opens in response to swallowing to allow food to enter the stomach. When you are not swallowing, this lower esophageal sphincter is tightly closed and prevents stomach contents such as hydrochloric acid and constituents of the bile from flowing backward into the lower esophagus (gastroesophageal reflux). In some individuals, either in response to a hernia of the stomach that protrudes into the chest along the lower esophagus (hiatus hernia), heredity or aging, the sphincter becomes incompetent and opens during rest. It opens further if intra-abdominal pressure is increased during straining, stooping or lifting heavy objects, or during pregnancy. Reflux is always worse within one hour of eating, especially if excess fluids were taken. A high-fat meal delays emptying of the stomach, and reflux may last for hours rather than minutes. The reflux of acid and stomach contents such as pepsin, bile salts and pancreatic enzymes causes severe irritation and at times inflammation of the lower esophagus. The condition is called an esophagitis, which is similar to having an ulcer in the stomach. Distressing symptoms persist for many years and may result in narrowing (stricture) of the lower esophagus with difficulty in swallowing.

Reflux esophagitis commonly causes discomfort in the lower chest (retrosternal) as does heart attack or angina. The burning, pressure-like pain or discomfort can radiate along the entire breastbone to the back and sometimes the arm. Heartburn is common, and regurgitation of bitter sour fluid or food, without vomiting, commonly occurs. Free acid reflux in the esophagus when an individual is sleeping can cause that person to be awakened by the discomfort. Spicy and acid foods, especially citrus juice, coffee and fatty meals increase the discomfort, which at times may be difficult to differentiate from a heart condition such as angina.

As mentioned earlier, a heart attack commonly causes profuse sweating and shortness of breath, whereas reflux esophagitis does not. The ECG remains normal when pain originates from the esophagus or stomach.

The diagnosis is made by X-ray. Using a barium swallow or a meal, the radiologist documents reflux of barium from the stomach into the esophagus. Tests are available to detect incompetence of the cardiac sphincter, and gastroscopy shows inflammation of the lower end of the esophagus with or without the presence of a hiatus hernia. A hernia often increases reflux, but the effect is variable. Reflux commonly occurs without the presence of hernia and may not occur when a hernia is present.

Esophageal reflux is relieved by:

- Taking antacids.
- Elevating the head of the bed and refraining from lying down for at least two hours after a meal or a drink of liquid.
- Avoiding spicy foods, fatty foods and acid liquids such as citrus juices.
- Avoiding bending, stooping and lifting, especially within one hour after meals.
- Reducing weight.
- Using drugs such as metoclopramide, which increases the tone or competence of the lower esophageal sphincter (see Fig. 5).

Esophageal Spasm

This condition is not as common as gastroesophageal reflux, but can closely mimic a heart attack and frequently occurs in patients who have esophageal reflux. It can occur at any age but is more common after age 40. The most common site of pain is behind the lower half of the breastbone and can radiate upward along the breastbone to the throat, jaw, back or arms. Pain can be squeezing, dull or sharp; moderate to severe; and last minutes to hours. The pain can occur at night, the individual being awakened by moderately severe pain that can be mistaken for a heart attack. Pain may come on during or after a meal, especially after a drink of cold liquid. Severe anxiety and stress can produce an attack, but there may be no precipitating factors.

In many patients with esophageal spasm, there is some difficulty in swallowing, and this can occur with or without the presence of pain. The diagnosis is usually confirmed by X-ray fluoroscopy during which the individual swallows liquid barium. Other confirmatory tests can be done by a gastroenterologist. Nitroglycerin may relieve the pain of esophageal spasm. As well, a calcium antagonist, nifedipine, which relieves muscle spasm, can sometimes abolish the pain of esophageal spasm. Antacids or warm milk may relieve the pain of esophageal spasm, but not the pain of heart attack. An ECG done when pain is present is normal and excludes a heart attack.

Lung Infections

Pneumonia may produce pain, and this is usually a sharp pain that is made worse by taking a very deep breath or coughing. The pain occurs because the outer membrane of the lung, the pleura, is involved in the inflammation, that is, a pleurisy. Usually there are fever, chills and cough.

Pericarditis

This is an inflammation of the outer membrane of the heart, which can be caused by a virus or bacteria, or may occur a few days after a heart attack. The pain is usually sharp, located over the lower breastbone or a little to the left of the breastbone, and is sometimes made worse by deep breathing when the pericardium and pleura are both involved. The pain is usually made worse by lying down and is improves within seconds or minutes on sitting up and leaning forward. Three or four days after a heart attack, a few patients develop pericarditis. This resolves in a few days. There are many other causes of pericarditis: kidney failure, cancer, lupus, radiation and as side effects of drugs.

Chest Wall Pain

Pain occurring in the wall of the chest is extremely common and may be due to pain in the muscles, ribs and costochondral joints. A costochondral joint is formed at a point where the hard bone of the rib joins the softer bone (cartilage) that attaches to the breastbone. The costochondral joints frequently get an irritation termed a costochondritis. Pain can be localized to a small area the size of one or two fingertips and the area is tender to pressure. Sitting in a draft or exercise such as raking a lawn may aggravate the condition. Costochondritis is very common between the ages of 30 and 60, and occasionally patients may become worried that it is the heart; the condition is much more common in women and occurs more often on the left side over the second and third costochondral joints. The pain is usually relieved by pain medications such as aspirin, but can recur over several months. The doctor may inject the joint with a combination of a local anesthetic and a cortisone compound, and this causes relief for several months, during which time nature heals the condition. The pain may return some time in the next few years. The important thing is to understand that it is a benign condition that never gets worse and does not lead to heart attacks or arthritis in other parts of the body. We must emphasize, however, that in a few patients, costochondritis can coincide with heart pain.

Arm Pain, Tingling and Numbness

Many people experience tingling and numbness in the arm if the arm is rested over the back of a chair for several minutes or hours, or by sleeping on the arm in an unusual position. This pain is caused by pressure on the nerve, and normally subsides quickly once the unusual pressure has been removed. Arm pain, tingling and numbness may occur when the nerves supplying the upper limb become affected by conditions such as arthritis of the spine in the neck region. Pressure is then exerted on the roots of the nerves as they emerge from the spine. Cervical disc disease is similar to the common condition, sciatica, which produces low back and leg pain. Pain arising from the above condition usually lasts several hours and may occur over many days and may be related to posture. As well, it is an aching pain and is only occasionally associated with chest pain. Nerve and muscle pain does not get worse during vigorous walking. This serves to differentiate the pain from angina, which can cause pain in the arm during brisk walking. Moderate to severe pain in the wrist or the arm without trauma or other precipitating cause, especially if there is no tenderness on pressure or movement of the limb, warrants medical advice.

AMBULANCE

If you think you are experiencing the symptoms and signs of a heart attack (see Heart Attack Signs and Symptoms) you should get to the hospital emergency room as quickly as possible. Denial or wishful thinking that the pain will disappear in the next hour is about the worst thing you can do. Do not try to reach a physician for advice. Call the ambulance first, then ask someone make a call to your doctor or cardiologist. If you can't reach the doctor, leave a message; do not wait for a reply. If you are fortunate to live in an area where a mobile heart ambulance exists, then please use this service. If this is not available, use 911 or ambulance service. If no ambulances are available, have someone drive you immediately to an emergency room. DO NOT DRIVE YOURSELF TO THE HOSPITAL if you have pain lasting longer than 15 minutes, particularly if you have unusual profuse sweating, shortness of breath, dizziness or feel weak.

While waiting for the ambulance, which should arrive within minutes of your call, try to keep calm. Fear and panic cause further damage to the heart because they provoke the secretion of adrenaline, which increases the work of the heart and may increase the size of the heart attack or induce abnormal heart rhythms. While waiting, do the following:

- Chew and swallow one 325-mg plain aspirin immediately.
- Do not take a coated aspirin because it takes several hours to be effective. Any form of regular aspirin (Bayer, Alka-Seltzer) may suffice to prevent a heart attack.
- Sit or lie propped up on three or four pillows and take a nitroglycerin tablet under the tongue. One tablet can do no harm. It will help calm your nerves as it will increase the blood supply to the coronary arteries. It also pools blood in the veins of the legs; therefore, less blood returns to the heart so there is less work for it to do. Nitroglycerin may decrease the size of a heart attack. It is reassuring to take one tablet under the tongue and believe that it will help. The drug is not as effective if you are lying flat. It is most effective if you sit up with your legs dangling over the edge of the bed or in a comfortable chair; this causes the blood to stay in the legs longer. Nitroglycerin may cause a headache, but this is to be expected because the drug dilates arteries, including those in the scalp as well as the coronary arteries.

There is no need to worry about the throbbing that you will feel in the head. The drug does not increase blood pressure.

- Put on a pajama top or loose shirt or blouse. Do not over-dress. There is no reason to put on a vest, sweater, shirt, tie, jacket or blouse that is difficult to remove. The garments will only have to be pulled off when you are in pain and lying on a stretcher in the emergency room. Therefore, if it is not excessively cold, wear clothing that can be easily opened to allow the doctor to examine you quickly and facilitate place-ment of the leads of the electrocardiogram (ECG, EKG) that must go on the chest. In addition, blood pressure is best taken with no garment around the arm. Every ambulance should have blankets to keep you warm. To re-emphasize, it is a waste of precious time to try to remove clothing in the emergency room.

When the ambulance arrives, you will be given oxygen. Oxygen given at this stage will help allay anxiety and panic. It is certainly helpful during the few minutes' wait. Put the oxygen mask right over your nose and mouth and breathe in the gas. There is nothing like believing that something will help when you are scared to death. We strongly recommend the use of oxygen and nitroglycerin as a technique to break the fear-anxiety-adrenaline reaction.

The reassurance of a trusted physician or specialist and the use of morphine can be lifesaving. Until these are avail-able, use aspirin, nitroglycerin and oxygen. They will help. Someone telling you to stay calm during the pain and fear of a heart attack is of no avail. Therefore, do the things that carry some hope. Remember, too, morphine is used not only to relieve pain but to relieve anxiety. Morphine is the best drug for this purpose, and you should not be opposed to its use. If a second injection is necessary, even if your pain is mild, do not object to the physician's using a second or several doses of morphine.

Mobile Coronary Care Ambulance

When a plaque of atheroma ruptures, a clot is formed within min-utes. This causes centrally located chest pain associated with sweating and often shortness of breath. If you believe you are having a heart attack, quickly go to the emergency room of the nearest hospital. Approximately 500,000 individuals with heart attacks die each year in the U.S. and Canada before reaching the hospital. The only way to save some of these lives is by the use of mobile heart squads. It is estimated that about 50,000 lives could be saved annually in North America by the use of heart squads.

The first mobile coronary care ambulances were operated at the Royal Victoria Hospital in Belfast by Dr. J. F. Pantridge and Dr. J. S. Geddes in 1965. The objective was to reach the patient quickly and stabilize the heart rhythm, relieve pain, as well as to afford reassurance and thus prevent death from abnormal heart rhythms. When the heart is found to be quivering and not contracting (ventricular fibrillation), the heart is defibrillated using a portable defibrillator. The success of such units led to the establishment of coronary care ambulances in Seattle and several other U.S. cities.

During 1972, one of the authors tried to establish a mobile coronary care ambulance in Ottawa. Hospital approval to bypass the emergency room and take patients directly to the coronary care unit was successful. After many months of stressful organizing and lobbying, the expected government grant support did not materialize. The government hoped at that time to give consideration to such projects during the early 1980s; however, we must emphasize that in the late 1990s, properly equipped emergency care ambulances are still lacking in Canada and in many areas of the United States. Perhaps with the advent of the new drugs that dissolve clots in the coronary arteries and the emphasis on early administration of such treatment for success, special mobile units may become necessary if we wish to save the countless lives lost before reaching hospitals.

To re-emphasize, in North America about half a million deaths occur outside the hospital whereas about 60,000 die from a heart attack in the hospital. It is estimated that coronary care units save about 30,000 to 40,000 lives annually in North America, at a very high but justifiable cost of running such units.

It is simple to equip and run mobile emergency care units. The vital equipment consists of a lightweight portable defibrillator, an ECG recorder, intravenous preparations, morphine and oxygen. A system in a city of one million people can be serviced by two units at a cost of about $100,000. It is the manpower that escalates the cost of running such units. It is feasible to send out a trained physician, a nurse and a driver trained in cardiopulmonary resuscitation in such a unit. Perhaps doctors in training will see the need for such services in a community and help to organize systems with the help of their chiefs and with financial assistance from service clubs until government bodies are made aware of the life-saving potential that justifies the cost of mobile emergency care units.

We would hope that by 1999, the drugs to dissolve clots in the coronary artery may prove useful and safe to be given, intravenously, by trained staff running mobile heart squads.

The public can assist by lobbying their elected representatives to achieve better mobile emergency care services. We can fly to the moon but, alas, we cannot save millions for lack of a simple application of common sense.

DRUGS TO DISSOLVE CLOTS

Four drugs have been shown to be successful in dissolving clots in the coronary artery: streptokinase, tissue-type plasminogen activator (tPA), reteplase and anistreplase (APSAC).

Streptokinase has been shown to be useful when infused directly through an arm vein, and it dissolves the clot in about 60 percent of patients. The drugs must be given within four hours of the onset of symptoms to be successful, but some benefit is seen up to six hours. Streptokinase, tPA, reteplase or APSAC given intravenously through an arm vein have a 70 percent chance of dissolving a clot in the coronary artery. An Italian clinical trial in 1986 and a UK trial in 1988 have shown intravenous streptokinase to be useful in preventing deaths in patients given the drug within four hours of onset of their heart attack. The beneficial effect is improved markedly when an aspirin is taken along with streptokinase. The drug tPA (alteplase) does not cause allergic reactions as seen occasionally with streptokinase. These reactions are, however, very mild and occur in less than 2 percent of patients. While tPA is slightly more effective than streptokinase, the cost is $2,000 versus $200. Although the benefits are mainly seen up to six hours from onset of symptoms, the timing has been extended to up to 12 hours after the onset of symptoms. There is great hope for patients who have suffered a heart attack provided they can get quickly to the emergency room of a hospital.

In some patients, after the clot is dissolved, it may be necessary two to three months later to crush the underlying plaque of atheroma with a special balloon catheter (see Angioplasty and Atheroma).

HOSPITALIZATION

If you still have pain on arrival at the emergency room, you can be reassured that the pain will be relieved within five minutes. Usually no time is wasted. The emergency room staff are primed to move quickly to deal with ambulance cases, in particular, those suspected to be heart attack victims. Thus, while your friend or your spouse gives your particulars, you are mainly expected to say to the nurse or the doctor that you are having chest pain. Point to the area of pain, indicating whether it is severe or very severe and that you are scared and would like something as soon as possible for the pain. You can then cooperate by answering all the other questions that the doctor may wish to ask. You will usually have to state whether you are allergic to medications. You will quickly receive an intravenous injection of morphine, which relieves the pain in two to five minutes. Since the injection is given intravenously, very small doses are used; for example, it may be given in 2-mg increments every minute until the pain is completely relieved.

Remember, do not be embarrassed to say that you are scared. A heart attack makes everyone afraid, and the doctor may sometimes forget this. Also, relief of pain by morphine can prevent some complications of a heart attack.

You will be quickly hooked up to continuous oxygen, and a blood pressure cuff will be placed around your arm. The doctor will examine you and ask you relevant questions. There is very little reason for the doctor to ask more than 12 questions, since the diagnosis is usually easily made from your description of the chest pain and from the ECG that is done within minutes of your arrival. The ECG writes the electrical rhythm and rate of each heartbeat. You will be immediately hooked up to a cardiac monitor: small electrodes similar to ECG electrodes are placed on your chest and these are connected to the monitor. The electrodes detect the electrical impulses from the heart, which are recorded continuously on a monitored screen. The nurses and doctors can see the visual display of the continuous electrocardiogram, showing each heartbeat as well as the important heart rate and rhythm of the heart. If the ECG confirms the diagnosis of heart attack, streptokinase, tPA or reteplase is given intravenously to dissolve the clot. In some hospitals with equipment and special staff, a coronary angiogram is done and angioplasty is used instead of drugs to clear the obstruction in the artery. This technique is life-saving but needs to be tested in large clinical trials.

The area of damaged muscle during a heart attack may cause electrical discharges that interrupt the normal clock-like rhythm of the heart, causing premature beats. These premature beats will show up on the monitor (see Palpitations). If these extra beats are frequent or of a special variety, they act as warning signals and the doctor suppresses these beats by giving a drug called lidocaine intravenously and then through a continuous intravenous drip. The drug is effective in stabilizing the heart rhythm and has no serious side effects, so you have no need to worry or be afraid.

We intend to give you reassuring news. It is important for you to start seeing the brighter side of things. Once the morphine is given, the worst is over. You are out of danger since you have made it to the hospital, where expert care is available. Most deaths occur before the patient reaches the hospital. Those who die before reaching the hospital have either a very large heart attack, experience electrical disturbances that cause the heart to quiver (ventricular fibrillation) or stop beating, or have remained too long outside of the hospital with extensive damage to the heart muscle.

Blood is taken and several blood tests are done; the ones that are necessary for the diagnosis are those for cardiac enzymes. The heart muscle cells that are deprived of blood undergo a series of changes ranging from injury to death of the cells and liberate three of these enzymes, which can be detected in the blood; the most reliable is the creatine kinase (CK). In some hospitals, the special fraction of CK (CKMB) that is derived solely from heart muscle is measured to distinguish it from the release from ordinary skeletal muscle. The ECG taken hourly for six hours then daily for a few days is the quickest, most reliable and least expensive test for detecting a heart attack.

The damaged heart muscle will heal itself over the next few weeks. Although it will be difficult, you should try not to worry about the future at this time. You need rest and reassurance; let others do the worrying.

Coronary Care Unit (CCU)

Hospitals that provide efficient heart care strive to get patients to the coronary care unit (CCU) within a half hour of emergency room arrival and soon after commencing streptokinase or tPA. The CCU is a special area of the hospital, usually six to 12 beds with a staff of specially trained doctors and nurses along with sophisti-cated electronic equipment to deal with heart attack patients. It will take some adjustment, over six to 24 hours, for a patient to get used to all the gadgets. The patient will have already had an ECG in the emergency room, and this is repeated in the CCU and once daily for three days. The patient is attached to a cardiac monitor similar to the one used in the emergency room.

The ECG is the main diagnostic tool and can accurately make the diagnosis in the majority of patients. In more than 90 percent of cases during a first heart attack, typical findings occur on the ECG and are easily recognized. If the first ECG is only suggestive of a heart attack, the repeat ECG six and 24 hours later usually gives an accurate diagnosis. In patients who have had previous heart attack, the ECG is less diagnostic and is positive in about 75 percent of the cases. To re-emphasize, less than 10 percent of patients having a first heart attack have an ECG that may not be diagnostic and it can be normal in about 5 percent of the cases. In these difficult cases, when the ECG is repeated six to 24 hours later, typical changes confirm or exclude the diagnosis of a heart attack.

It is necessary in a difficult case for the doctor in the emer-gency room to pay special attention to the patient's description of the chest discomfort. Therefore, in such cases, the patient must put up with answering questions posed by several doctors. Perhaps the fortunate patient is not having a heart attack. In this case, the doctor may elect to admit the individual for observation for 24 hours. The creatine kinase (CKMB), a cardiac enzyme, starts to increase about four to six hours after the heart attack and may be normal in some cases if tested for very early during the attack. A careful physician often repeats the ECG and blood test for CKMB every two hours. If both ECG and CKMB are normal and the description of chest pain does not suggest a heart attack, the doctor may elect to send the individual home after 24 hours. The patient is advised to return to the emergency room if the pain recurs. A risk is therefore taken and the public must understand that the doctor may not be able to admit every patient and that the pain may be due to other causes. Policy varies depending on the physician in charge. If doubt exists, the patient is admitted and if three ECGs done over a 48-hour period and a repeat test for cardiac enzymes is normal, then a heart attack can be excluded with confidence. In rare instances, the diagnosis is firmly established only on the third day of the illness.

A routine chest X-ray is given. It cannot diagnose a heart attack; it is useful in making the diagnosis of heart failure, which occurs for a few days in more than 50 percent of heart attack patients.

Occasionally the blood pressure is very low and drug combinations are given intravenously to maintain the systolic blood pressure between 90 and 100. Blood pressure of 95 to 105 systolic is very common in patients having heart attacks, but it can be 110 to 140 in those who had slightly higher blood pressure before the heart attack.

In some units, other instruments are used to monitor the amount of blood ejected from the left ventricle, that is, the cardiac output. Because of the many parameters that are measured, several veins in the arm may be used for the introduction of a venous tube, which is usually about one to two inches long and is not harmful.

An echocardiogram may be done to verify the strength of the heart muscle. Nuclear scans can be helpful in the few patients who do not have classical diagnostic findings on the electrocardiogram or cardiac enzymes. It is not routine to have nuclear scans because the ECG and blood test for cardiac enzymes are sufficient in more than 90 percent of the cases for a firm diagnosis. Nuclear scans and other tests increase the cost to both patient and state and are not justifiable.

In patients with a heart attack and complications such as severe heart failure, a monitoring catheter may be inserted into the right side of the heart to monitor the pressure within the heart; this assists with evaluation of the treatment in critically ill patients. If the patient is not critically ill and complications have not occurred, this expensive and invasive test is not justifiable.

The procedure for introducing the catheter is simple. The skin area over the vein is infiltrated with local anesthetic. The specially made fine tube (catheter) has a tiny balloon and sensing devices at its tip. The catheter is inserted into the vein and threaded into the right ventricle and the pulmonary artery. The position is verified by X-ray.

Patients with severe heart failure and very low blood pressure may require several drugs and fluid replacement given intravenously. The monitoring catheter that is positioned in the pulmonary artery is useful for the infusion of intravenous preparations, but a simple intravenous in the arm vein is preferable in the majority of cases, because this method is inexpensive and devoid of complications.

Day One. Treatment is continued with oxygen, which can be

discontinued after a few hours in the majority of patients. The amount of oxygen in the arterial blood is tested by a simple measurement, and if this is normal, the oxygen is usually discontinued, which is reassuring news.

Generally, no food or drink is allowed for the first eight hours, since the process of digestion steals blood from the heart; also, if vomiting occurs, vomitus may be aspirated into the lung.

During the stay in the coronary care unit, the patient receives sufficient sedation to prevent anxiety and to ensure adequate rest.

Day Two. A light diet is usually given and increased over a few days to a normal diet. On the second day, patients are usually sitting at the bedside.

Days Three to Five. Late on the second or on the third day, the patient is moved from the coronary care unit to an intermediate care area or to a ward with other patients. In the standard room, the patient is allowed more freedom each day starting with walks to the bathroom and progressing then by day five to walks in the corridor of the hospital. If the individual is making a good recovery, the intravenous tubes are removed by the third or fourth day. The education process will now begin and both husband and wife are usually given instructions together in a question and answer period each day. The individual is often concerned that pain is no longer present and wonders why it is necessary to stay in the hospital. The pain of a heart attack usually disappears between one and six hours, and in most patients, there is usually no recurrence of pain during the hospital stay and in many there is no pain for several years.

By the fourth day, the patient is very well and enjoys meals and walks around alone. At this stage the doctor will wish to discuss the question of how much rest is necessary. The patient must understand that a blockage of a coronary artery has taken place. This caused damage and death to a segment of heart muscle cells. Special cells in the body that form bridges (scar tissue cells) move into the area and form scar tissue joining the two normal areas of heart muscle. The scar tissue is similar to that following the healing of a surgical incision. It takes time for scar tissue to form and heal. The healing process usually takes three to six weeks. During the 1950s, it was common practice to keep patients in hospital for four to eight weeks. In the 1970s, it became apparent that after seven days, if there were no complications, most patients could be allowed home. In some countries discharge on the fourth or fifth day is not unusual.

In most hospitals, patients are discharged home between the sixth and 10th day depending on the size of infarction, complications, and their home situation.

Day Six. By the sixth day, the patient is walking approximately 100 feet, two or three times daily, and by the seventh to the 10th day, has been supervised while walking up one flight of stairs and may have had a stroll on the treadmill to reach a heart rate of 120 per minute. This modified stress test is repeated in six to 10 weeks and decisions are then made regarding further medical treatment, angioplasty or bypass surgery. The heart rhythm is usually checked for 24 hours using a Holter monitor to ensure that severe rhythm disturbances do not occur.

HEART ATTACK AND EMOTIONAL IMPACT

For most people, suffering a heart attack is a traumatic mental experience. Uncertainty about the financial impact, the work situation, relationships and in particular, sexual activity may cause depression and anxiety. Social workers, nurses and the medical team must find time to listen and talk to the patient. Explanations and answers must be clear so that the patient understands that, after a heart attack, a normal life is possible for the majority. The sophisticated gadgets of modern medicine cannot replace the reassuring words of an understanding, caring physician.

Reassurance is important not only to the patient but also to the patient's family. The patient's relative is often in distress and must receive adequate counseling from the nursing staff, medical health staff and the physician in charge. During the entire hospital stay, a few minutes spent each day with the relative to answer questions is most rewarding and greatly appreciated.

Depression and Anxiety

The majority of heart attack patients experience some degree of depression and anxiety. To combat this complication, both the doctor and the nurses must communicate with the patient in an open and frank manner so that the patient can air feelings and have all questions answered during his or her last seven days in the hospital. A social worker may have to be involved in some cases; supportive home visits, advice on job orientation and discussions regarding financial matters may be necessary. Discussions are necessary during the next three months; two weekly visits to an understanding family doctor may help to dissipate depression with the recognition that all is not lost. The doctor should reassure the patient that depression and anxiety with the associated weakness and tiredness are normal and will be alleviated with time. It takes six weeks for the damaged muscle to heal and form a firm scar. During the same six weeks, anxiety and depression dissipate in the majority of patients. The first four weeks will be tough. Thereafter, the assistance of an exercise program, the ability to drive again, and the return of sexual activity help to remove despair. Time heals all wounds, including the muscle damage and psychological insults. A few (less than 1 percent of patients) require antidepressant drugs. They are nonaddicting and can be very useful when given as a single bedtime dose for three to a maximum of 12 weeks. An exercise rehabilitation program is useful in many respects and is of definite assistance in the management of most heart attack patients.

DIET AFTER A HEART ATTACK

A low-salt diet is prescribed only for patients with heart failure who require water pills (diuretics) or the heart pill digoxin, as well as for the previously hypertensive patient (see Table 3). Patients are advised on the use of a weight reduction diet and a modified diet to reduce cholesterol and saturated fat intake. Lipid-lowering drugs may be considered for patients who have LDL cholesterol greater than 100 mg (2.5 mmol).

The total cholesterol, LDL and HDL cholesterol are estimated for the patient in the hospital and three months later. The goal is to maintain the LDL cholesterol at less than 100 mg (2.5 mmol) (see Heart Attack Prevention Diet). Alcohol should be avoided for the first four weeks; thereafter one to two ounces daily are allowed. Alcohol is restricted if heart failure is present or if the heart is enlarged.

REHABILITATION, RETIREMENT AND TRAVEL

Most patients under age 65 can return to work between six and 12 weeks after discharge. The return date takes into account the patient's age, financial resources, existing diseases and type of work. The physical and emotional stress associated with the job should be thoroughly explored.

Patients with uncomplicated myocardial infarctions are advised to increase activity so as to return to about 90 percent of the pre-infarction level in three months. If at six to 10 weeks the exercise stress test and ejection fraction (the volume of blood the heart pumps) are satisfactory, your prognosis should be excellent. Types of exercise are discussed in Exercise and the Heart. Exercise at home is graduated as follows: During the first three days at home, walk in the house; for the remainder of the first week, walk outside the home 50 to 100 yards daily. The second week, walk 200 yards once or twice daily. The third week, cover 300 yards once or twice daily. The fourth week, go a quarter mile or 440 yards once or twice daily. During the fifth week, walk a half mile daily, and during the sixth week, one mile once or twice daily. This is a rough estimate of what you should be doing during the weeks after a heart attack. Thereafter, if you feel well and have no chest pain, you should be able to do much more exercise; this includes joining exercise programs. One- to three-mile walks are usual by the eighth week. Doubles tennis, golf and similar past times are reasonable at three months.

Patients may join supervised exercise programs provided there is no evidence of:

- Persistent heart failure
- Angina
- Abnormal heart rhythm such as frequent premature beats (see Palpitations)
- Moderate to severe problems with heart valves

A stress test is useful at some point, especially if you want to do further activities. In patients under age 70, a stress test done between the sixth and 10th week should result in the patient being able to do more than seven minutes of walking on the treadmill. Patients who can complete about nine minutes without undue shortness of breath, chest pain or ECG changes, which indicate oxygen lack to the heart muscle, are usually allowed to engage in all exercise activities. Competitive sports and extreme exertion should be avoided. Patients who can complete six minutes, but need to stop because of fatigue, tiredness or leg discomfort and who show a normal heart rate and blood pressure without an abnormal heart rhythm or ECG changes, are allowed to participate in a restricted and, if possible, supervised exercise program, but they should be retested in three months. Exercise programs should be individualized. There are many useful rehabilitation programs attached to major hospitals. Provided that adequate supervision is obtained, exercise programs play a great role in assisting patients to maintain good body tone and to return to participation in games, sexual activity and work they were accustomed to before a heart attack.

We strongly endorse exercise programs, provided that the patient is stress-tested and conditions that contraindicate exercise programs are reviewed by the physician for each individual. There is no evidence that moderate to strenuous exercise prevents heart attacks or limits the size of a heart attack. The physician should recognize the minority of patients in whom a very gradual program or only mild exercises are appropriate. Walking certainly provides safe and adequate exercise.

Because you have had a heart attack, it does not mean that you will be crippled for life. About 10 million North Americans can testify that you can recover from a heart attack and go on to live a very active and normal life. The majority return to the same job. Within three to six months, the majority engage in the same activities as prior to the heart attack. Tennis, golf and skiing are only a few of the many activities that are enjoyed. Some individuals lead a more active life and learn to handle stress and often report that they feel better than 10 years prior to their heart attack. If you like jogging, you should know that six months after their heart attack, more than 50 percent of patients are able to jog one to three miles daily. We are not suggesting that you do this, but if you enjoy jogging, then one to two miles four times weekly will improve your endurance. Similar exercises including a one- to three-mile walk and stair climbing are suitable activities.

Don'ts

- Do not do static exercises such as weightlifting or push-ups. Such exercise uses sustained muscular contraction that squeezes the blood vessels, and thus increases blood pressure and the work of the heart.
- Do not exercise immediately after a meal. Wait one to two hours after a light snack or two to three hours after a heavy meal.
- Do not exercise if you have a fever.

- Do not stop exercising suddenly; always warm up and cool down for five to 10 minutes.
- During the first six weeks at home, do not engage in strenuous exercise or housework such as heavy cleaning or repairs, gardening such as raking leaves or mowing the lawn, or snow shoveling.
- Do not take a hot or cold shower immediately before or after exercise. Do not take a sauna because the heat dilates the vessels in the skin and steals blood away from the heart and the brain.

Retirement

Retirement may well be a problem for many individuals, especially those who do not have enough hobbies to keep them sufficiently occupied. They become bored and depressed, and therefore retirement must be selective. If possible, it is best to get back to work since this prevents the development of neurosis and depression. There is no doubt that returning to a job that was previously distressing to the individual can lead to further harm. Patients who can afford to change jobs or retire and have enough hobbies do extremely well. The good news is that the disease may burn itself out. Individuals who have had large heart attacks with complications such as severe heart failure that restrict exercise programs are strongly advised to retire, especially if they are over 60. A change in lifestyle may be lifesaving.

Travel

Patients should not drive for about six weeks. If a stress test is satisfactory at three weeks, necessary flying is allowed. Otherwise elective flights should be postponed beyond three months. Patients with stable angina are allowed to fly any time, but not if angina is unstable (see Angina). Patients should take along a current ECG. This may save unnecessary admission to a hospital and provide a physician with a prior ECG for comparison. Nitroglycerin should be carried, too, along with all medications advised by the doctor. Oxygen is not necessary during the flight.

SEXUAL ACTIVITIES

Sex is a part of living. For the majority, it is one of the most enjoyable, satisfying, stress-relieving activities that life provides. Most of what is said relates to men because the heart attack rate is far more common in men than women at age 35 to 65. Also, men have far more hang-ups about sex than women, especially since a man cannot will an erection. Fear interferes with performance; thus some men, owing to a lack of proper discussion with their doctor before hospital discharge, develop fears that may cause problems with sexual function. In addition, the female partner develops fear and apprehension that intercourse could cause the death of her husband. The female partner may therefore turn the whole thing off. This disturbance in a marital relationship can be quite traumatic and increase the anxiety and depression that is so common after a heart attack.

It is important for males to understand that a heart attack does not cause impotence, and that if you do not have intercourse for six weeks, it will not alter sexual performance in the future. The good news is that 12 weeks after a heart attack, more than 75 percent of patients are able to engage in sexual intercourse with the same frequency as before. To re-emphasize, a heart attack is not the end of your sex life. Some physicians believe that sex can be resumed about two weeks after discharge from the hospital. But the majority of physicians agree that it is reasonable and safe to resume intercourse about six weeks after a heart attack. There is no hard-and-fast rule; you should do what comes naturally and without fear. If, about four weeks after discharge, you are able to walk one mile and climb two flights of stairs without chest discomfort or undue shortness of breath and experience the urge to have sex with your usual partner, then you should go ahead without fear of precipitating another heart attack.

The amount of physical exertion required during sexual intercourse is equivalent to walking up about four flights of stairs or a brisk one-mile walk. Most heart attack patients should be engaging in this type of exercise about six weeks after a heart attack. If during such activity there is no chest discomfort or undue shortness of breath, sexual activities are considered safe. In a study of 6,000 cases of sudden death, only 34 were related to sexual intercourse and 27 of those deaths occurred during extramarital sexual relations. Sudden death or heart attack is extremely rare when the heart attack patient engages in intercourse with the usual partner. Most deaths in males during intercourse occur while engaging with partners other than their wives. Middle-aged males who have been married for a number of years are at greatest risk. Intercourse with a much younger extramarital female partner may lead to more emotional reactions, causing a much higher increase of blood pressure and heart rate, thus putting the heart under severe strain. Furthermore, such a relation may also be accompanied by the ingestion of a large meal and alcohol, which adds to cardiac work.

It is advisable to use the position to which you are most accustomed. There is no reason to change to side to side or female on top if this was not the most often practiced and most favorable position. If the patient is male and erection is easily achieved, the female on top — superior crouched — is often recommended. In this position, the woman has both knees touching the bed for traction. Therefore, she is the active partner. What is most familiar is always the best position as it increases confidence in the male and allays anxiety in the female, who is afraid that the husband may die or have a heart attack during intercourse.

There is no need to decrease the frequency of sexual activity. To re-emphasize, after three months if there is no chest pain, undue shortness of breath or palpitations on walking two to three miles or climbing four flights of stairs or jogging one mile, the individual should be capable of enjoying the same sexual frequency as before the heart attack.

Don'ts

These apply to the first three months after a heart attack and for patients with chest pain on effort (angina) or heart failure:

- Do not take a hot shower immediately before intercourse. Hot showers or saunas dilate vessels of the skin, thus stealing blood from the heart and the brain.
- Do not have intercourse immediately after a heavy meal; wait two to three hours.
- Do not have more than one drink of alcohol or beer and indulge in intercourse. More than three drinks consumed in two hours will make it more difficult to achieve an erection and may also decrease heart muscle contraction.
- Smoking can also decrease sexual performance. Smoking has

been shown to cause constriction of small penile arteries and therefore impotence.

Suggestions

- A simple exercise program improves physical endurance and nearly always increases sexual performance. Therefore, start your walking program one week after discharge and increase it to a brisk one- to two-mile walk daily by the sixth week. Each week increase from one, then two, then three flights of stairs by the sixth week. If your hospital or community offers a rehabilitation program, it is wise to join this with the advice of your cardiologist. Or plan your own program with some common sense (see Heart Attack Rehabilitation). At this stage, you should know how to take your pulse and try to keep the heart rate for about five minutes within the target zone, i.e., 60 to 70 percent of your maximal heart rate (Table 2). After a few months of exercise, if you feel well, you can keep the heart rate in the target zone for about five to 10 minutes during 30 minutes of exercise. A stress test at this stage may increase your confidence, and your physician can advise on additional exercises.

- Rest is more important before rather than after sexual activity, although if you feel tired after the activity and feel like sleeping, certainly it is wise to have a half- to one-hour rest. Therefore, if possible, have intercourse in the morning after a night of sleep or any other time after rest or relaxation.

- If you are very short of breath or develop chest discomfort during intercourse, stop and take nitroglycerin. Discomfort during your first sexual relations does not mean the discomfort may occur again. It does not indicate that you are likely to develop a heart attack during intercourse. However, if pain does occur again or if there is any difficulty with sexual activity, be sure to discuss this with your doctor at the next office visit, which is usually about six weeks after discharge. Medications given on discharge may interfere with sexual performance, and these may be reduced at your next office visit. In particular, diuretics (water pills) and less commonly, beta-blockers, antihypertensive drugs or antidepressants can alter sexual performance. Patients who have angina and get pain on intercourse can get relief with beta-blockers, or 5 mg isosorbide dinitrate placed under the tongue 10 minutes prior to intercourse.

BETA-BLOCKERS

Beta-blocking drugs were discussed earlier (see Angina) and the present discussion explains mainly the rationale for their use in patients after a heart attack. Beta-blockers block the action of adrenaline and noradrenaline at receptor sites on the surface of cells. They cause a reduction in heart rate; therefore, less oxygen is required by the weakened heart muscle. They decrease the force of contraction of the heart muscles, and this further decreases the work and the amount of oxygen required by the heart. Most of the effects on the heart and arteries are related to this blocking of the actions of stress hormones. Beta-blockers stabilize the heart rhythm and can prevent premature beats, in particular, those that are precipitated by mental and physical stress. They can prevent some episodes of ventricular fibrillation, which is the cause of sudden death.

We must re-emphasize that beta-blockers, statins to lower cholesterol and aspirin are the only oral drugs that are proven by studies to prevent death from heart attacks. When beta-blockers are given to patients from about the seventh day after a heart attack and for two years, they significantly reduce the incidence of death from heart attack including sudden death. They also reduce the recurrent rate of subsequent heart attacks. About 70 of every 100 heart patients are eligible for treatment with beta-blockers and these include patients who have angina after the heart attack.

In the United Kingdom, a survey of actively practicing British consulting cardiologists was carried out to determine their practices when prescribing beta-blockers after a heart attack. Half of the cardiologists reported that they use beta-blockers in all patients who can take the drug starting about one week after the heart attack and continuing for about two years. The other half reported that they gave the beta-blockers to patients at high risk. We strongly recommend a beta-blocker to all post-heart attack patients from day seven if there is no contraindication to their use.

Despite the proven beneficial effects of beta-blockers, less than 33 percent of patients receive beta-blockers from their mighty physicians. About 50 percent of the physicians in North America are reluctant to prescribe the drugs for patients after a heart attack. This reluctance stems from the teaching of a minority of experts and failure to update their knowledge. The argument of the physicians who oppose the routine use of beta-blockers is as follows: Although the beta-blocker timolol has been shown to cause a 33 percent reduction in cardiac deaths and a 67 percent reduction in sudden deaths in a well-run multicenter randomized clinical trial, a 33 percent reduction means that of every 100 patients with a heart attack treated with a beta-blocker, "only" three lives can be saved. That is, if you take 100 heart attack patients discharged from hospital, studies have established that 10 patients will die in the next year; 33 percent of the 10 deaths can be saved — three patients. Thus these physicians believe that it is not worthwhile to treat 100 patients with a beta-blocker to save "only" three. Some physicians use expensive, sophisticated tests to determine high-risk patients who are likely to die in the next year. Beta-blockers are then given to the few patients who are termed high-risk. Prediction by tests, especially stress tests, nuclear scans and Holter monitoring, can be misleading, however.

To these opposing physicians, we pose the following question: The next 20 years of extensive and expensive research may produce a medication capable of a 60 percent reduction in deaths in patients who have had a heart attack and then treated for one year. This result will be accepted by all physicians as good news. If the majority of physicians will then agree to treat 100 to save six, why not treat 100 to save three at present? Is the difference between six and three that great? The new drugs for dissolving blood clots soon after a heart attack save two to five lives in every 100 patients treated and this is considered a major achievement. Logical therapeutic decision making and application of common sense in prescribing proven remedies appear to be a worldwide weakness of physicians.

The dose of a beta-blocker used for the prevention of death and recurrent heart attacks is not high and side effects are infrequent. A fall in pulse rate from the usual average 70 per minute to 55 per minute is expected if the drug is working. On mild to moderate exercise the heart rate stays under 120 per minute as opposed to racing to 140 to 150 with a moderate amount of exercise. The slowing of the pulse is a good effect; therefore, do not be afraid of a heart rate of 50 to 60 per minute. Only a few patients, less than 10 percent, get symptoms of dizziness if the pulse falls below 50 per minute. The dose of drug is then reduced by half and the pulse stabilizes between 54 and 64 per minute. In a few patients, the drug has to be discontinued because too much slowing may occur on a very small dose. Fortunately these sensitive patients are rare (less than 1 percent).

The commonly used beta-blocking drugs are:

- Timolol: 5 mg twice daily for a few weeks then 10 mg twice daily.
- Propranolol: 40 mg twice daily for two weeks then 80 mg twice daily for one month followed by 160 to 240 mg long-acting once daily in nonsmokers.
- Metoprolol: 50 mg twice daily for two weeks then 100 mg twice daily or Toprol XL, 50 to 100 mg once daily, is a major advance. The drug is unfortunately not available in Canada.
- Atenolol: 50 to 75 mg daily. A 25-mg tablet is available in the United States and is useful in the elderly.

Many other beta-blockers are available, but the ones listed have been shown to be useful in post-heart attack patients. Propranolol may not confer protection in smokers. It is important, therefore, to also discontinue smoking.

If you notice side effects, especially wheezing, increased shortness of breath, dizziness or impotence, reduce the daily dose by half and consult your doctor. Do not stop the drug suddenly. Impotence is very rare but does occur. The incidence is about four in every 100 patients treated. As emphasized, heart attacks do not cause impotence but can decrease sexual activity; therefore it may not be the drug. In any event, alteration in sexual activity should prompt the doctor to reduce the dose of beta-blocking drugs. If there is no improvement, the drug may be discontinued. The effect on sexual function is quickly reversible.

The use of beta-blocking drugs can save between 40,000 and 100,000 lives annually in the United States and Canada and, as well, many nonfatal heart attacks can be prevented. This information has been available since 1981. We trust that physicians would smarten up!

CASE HISTORY OF HEART PATIENT

O.W., age 47, was sitting watching television when he suddenly felt a pain in the center of his chest. The pain felt like nothing he had ever experienced before. The entire lower two-thirds of his breastbone and part of his left chest felt as if someone was crushing him in a vice. He started to feel weak and afraid, and he loosened his collar to relieve the feeling of strangulation. He called his wife for some antacid for what he assumed must be terrible indigestion due to the high-fat meal he had eaten 30 minutes earlier. Two antacid tablets did not relieve the pain and he started to pace restlessly around the room. He soon became dizzy, felt faint and was forced to lie down. The pain was not relieved by lying flat, so his wife propped him up and started rubbing his back. About seven to 10 minutes went by and the pain was becoming worse; he felt as if he was going to die. Though a sense of panic was beginning to set in, he did not want to alarm his wife. His entire life seemed to float before him. He was determined to sit up and to walk to see if it would ease the pain. He moved across the room; the dizziness was less than before, but the pain was of the same intensity. Both arms, from the shoulders to below the elbows, were now aching as if he carried a 50-pound weight in each hand. There was no pain in his back. He tried to analyze what could be the reason for this pain. He had not done any physical work in the past month. It could easily be stomach upset since there was some discomfort at the lower end of his breastbone and stomach (epigastric area). He had been under pressure at work for the last month. His job was on the line and he was determined to show his colleagues and boss that he could cope. He had faced similar stressful situations before. Suddenly, as he was wondering about the past, the pain became excruciating, constricting his chest. He could no longer hide his fear; his wife noticed his face had become pale. She dashed for the phone and called an ambulance, which came 20 minutes later. The wait was agonizing as his breathing and strangling sensation worsened. He had no nitroglycerin in the house since he was not known to have coronary heart disease. As soon as the ambulance arrived, an oxygen mask was applied and he was rushed to the emergency room of the nearest hospital. A diagnosis of an acute myocardial infarction was made and he was admitted to the coronary care unit of our hospital. He made a reasonable recovery and was discharged on the 10th hospital day. He did have mild heart failure during the first two days in the hospital but this cleared quickly. A few days after his attack, he was placed on a beta-blocker, propranolol, and a drug to try to prevent blood clotting, sulfinpyrazone. He discontinued his two-pack-a-day smoking habit. His cholesterol was 1.3 mmol (280 mg), that is, moderately elevated. He was not overweight but he was placed on a diet with low cholesterol and low saturated fat; moderate salt restriction was appropriate. He was placed on an exercise program. He had liked jogging in the past, and three months after his heart attack, he was able to jog one to three miles daily.

He did well for the next two years, during which time he took his medications regularly. He continued his exercise program doing three to 10 miles daily, six days weekly. About 18 months later, while standing in line at the bank he suddenly dropped to the floor. Fortunately, a trained nurse was in the line, and cardiopulmonary resuscitation was commenced. He was resuscitated and rushed to the hospital. He was found to have complete heart block, and a permanent pacemaker was inserted. He was discharged from the hospital a few days later and resumed his daily exercises.

About one year later, while on vacation, he suddenly experienced central chest pain that was similar to his first heart attack; he was rushed to the hospital. His attack was complicated by heart failure. His heart failure was cleared by the use of digoxin, a water pill, furosemide and a vasodilator called captopril. Investigations showed that he had developed an aneurysm, a small swelling of part of the heart muscle.

He wanted to get back on an exercise program. Though at this stage he was not the best candidate for exercise, he started slowly over the next few weeks by walking one to three miles. He eased into jogging a quarter mile daily, but when he tried to do a half mile, he started getting shortness of breath and pain in the chest. This pain was immediately relieved by stopping the run. Angina was present and he now agreed to have a catheter study. Coronary arteriography was done, and this showed a complete block in one artery, more than 80 percent obstruction in two branches and a small aneurysm of the left ventricle. He underwent coronary artery bypass surgery with three bypass grafts and repair of the aneurysm. Two weeks later, he was discharged from the hospital. He slowly began an exercise program, and 10 months later he was once again jogging one to two miles daily. He completed the Terry Fox 10 km Fun Run in September 1985 and 1990; in the late 1990s he enjoys a normal lifestyle.

RISK FACTORS AND PREVENTION

The identification of factors that increase the risk of heart attack has been made possible by various population studies, including the well-known Framingham Study. The statistical correlation has been so consistent as to enable researchers to state with confidence that high blood cholesterol, high blood pressure (hypertension) and cigarette smoking are major risk factors and, if present, increase your probability of having a fatal or nonfatal heart attack or stroke.

The risk factors can be subdivided into three groups:

Group I: Uncontrollable Risk Factors
1. Heredity. A strong family history of heart attack especially before age 55 increases the risk.
2. Age. Risk increases with age.
3. Sex. Everyone recognizes that heart attacks are about 10 times more common in men than in women in the 30-to-50 age group. After menopause and beyond age 70 women catch up.

Group II: Controllable Risk Factors
1. High blood cholesterol
2. Hypertension
3. Cigarette smoking
4. Stress

Group III: Other Factors of Importance
1. Diabetes
2. Sedentary lifestyle, lack of exercise
3. Strenuous unaccustomed exertion
4. Obesity
5. Type A personality

High blood pressure (hypertension) is a preventable risk factor. It is extremely difficult to get the population at risk to discontinue smoking. Hypertension, however, can be detected and does respond to nondrug treatment, and where this fails, safe and effective drugs are now available (see Hypertension).

It is well established that hypertension increases the risk of heart attacks, especially if there is concomitant high blood cholesterol and/or cigarette smoking. Hypertension causes mechanical damage to the lining of the artery, and cholesterol is drawn into the injured tissues.

There is conclusive scientific evidence that control of hypertension markedly lowers the incidence of stroke, heart failure and kidney damage, and it is believed to decrease the incidence of fatal and nonfatal heart attacks. Hypertension accelerates atherosclerosis; blockage or rupture of an artery occurs from 10 to 20 years earlier than in individuals with normal blood pressures.

In recent years, heart attacks have been observed in males age 27 to 34 but this occurrence is rare. Such males usually have a very high blood cholesterol, hypertension or rare diseases of the coronary arteries and a family history of heart attack before age 50. Heart attacks before age 27 are extremely rare and may occur in patients with familial hypercholesterolemia who have a cholesterol in the range of 600 to 1,000 mg (15 to 25 mmol). Menstruating females are often protected from heart attacks, except those who smoke and simultaneously take the birth control pill, or those with diabetes, hypertension and rare familial hypercholesterolemia. The family history is important. Individuals with a strong family history, that is, a parent and one or more uncles or aunts dying of heart attacks before age 55, have an increased risk. These individuals should have a medical checkup, including total cholesterol, LDL (bad) cholesterol and HDL ("good") cholesterol measurements at about age 25. The advice of a physician is required if the LDL is less than 4 mmol and HDL is less than 1 mmol. A stress test at about age 40 is appropriate if the cholesterol is borderline.

If you are a male over age 35 and have one of the four major risk factors — high blood cholesterol, hypertension, cigarette smoking or stress — your chance of having a heart attack doubles. Two risk factors increases your risk to more than three times that of a person with no risk factors. If you have all four and your mother or father had a heart attack prior to age 55, your risk increases to about seven times. No one can predict with any degree of certainty who is going to have a heart attack. Some people are just plain lucky. They have the correct genes; "they chose their parents." They disobey all the rules: two eggs and two packets of cigarettes daily from age 20 to 75, never exercise and lead a stressful life and yet never have a heart attack. People of this type are not overweight, and fortunately have blood pressures that are on the low side of normal (110 to 120 systolic). If your blood pressure is low (less than 120/80), and you are average or slightly underweight and your parents both lived to beyond 75, you are on the right side of the track. Women are at risk after age 55 and need preventive measures from at least age 48 (see Women and Heart Disease).

HEART ATTACK PREVENTION DIET

Consult Table 1 and follow the advice given in A, B and C below. This will fulfill the recommendation of fat intake to be 30 percent of food energy. You will receive enough polyunsaturated fat and protein without having to do complicated calculations. The American Heart Association Prudent Diet gives similar recommendations.

These recommendations do not strictly apply if your blood cholesterol is less than 200 mg (5 mmol) since you obviously deal with cholesterol by your own natural process. Foods with a high salt (sodium) content should be avoided or used sparingly. See Table 3.

    A. Do not use the following foods:
- Organ meats such as liver, kidney, sweetbreads, heart or brain.
- Meat fat, heavily marbled steaks, mutton, salt pork or duck.
- Whole milk or whole milk products, cream, lard and non-vegetable margarine, or vegetable margarine that has saturated fats or palm oil.
- Coconut oil or products containing coconut oil such as nondairy coffee cream substitutes, palm oil and peanut oil or peanut butter.

    B. Use the following foods sparingly and in small amounts:
- Roast beef, luncheon meats, bacon, sausages, hamburger and spare ribs.
- Butter, egg yolk, cheese made from whole milk or cream, pies, chocolate pudding, whole milk pudding and ice cream.
- Lobster, which has a high cholesterol content and is often served with abundant butter.
- Peanuts, cashews and brazil nuts.

    C. Use the following recommended foods often:
- All root vegetables; lentils and split peas, which are rich in protein and fiber; fruits daily including avocado despite its very small saturated fat content. Do not "overindulge" in vegetables containing a high content of vitamin K such as broccoli, alfalfa, turnip greens, squash and lettuce, because

an increase in vitamin K intake may increase clot formation.

- Fish of all types, even when described as fatty fish, contains little saturated fat but has an abundance of omega-3 fatty acids that protect the arteries. Shrimps are not as bad as claimed, provided they are not fried in batter and are used only occasionally. Remember, any food fried in batter increases the saturated fat content.
- Poultry, chicken breast, and turkey, which, when cooked with the skin off, contain little saturated fat or cholesterol. You must cut fat from meat, including chicken, before cooking.
- Lean beef or veal.
- Fat and oils: polyunsaturated vegetable oils with alpha-linolenic acid such as canola and soybean oil should be used for cooking, and polyunsaturated or olive oil margarine to be used as much as possible in place of butter. A margarine with added alpha-linolenic acid and without hydrogenation or added palm oil would be useful.
- Carbohydrates (sugars and starchy foods) such as bread or other flour products, potato and rice to maintain normal body weight.
- Onions and garlic. Use garlic powder, not garlic salt, which has a high sodium content (see Table 3).
- Alpha-linolenic acid: Walnuts and purslane are rich in alpha-linolenic acid and are strongly recommended. Alpha-linolenic acid is a long-chain fatty acid, which is a significant component of the Cretan Mediterranean diet. Alpha-linolenic acid has an aspirin-like effect and reduces the stickiness of blood platelets and thus prevents clotting in arteries. A clinical study using an alpha-linolenic acid–rich Mediterranean diet was reported in *Lancet*, June 1994, to be useful in decreasing recurrent heart attacks in patients following a first heart attack. The Mediterranean type diet consisted of: root and green vegetables, more bread, fish, poultry, less beef, lamb and pork; daily fruit, nuts, olive oil; butter was replaced by canola oil margarine with 5 percent alpha-linenolic acid added.

The Cretans and Japanese have the lowest heart attack mortality in the world and have a high intake of alpha-linolenic acid. The Cretans' source of alpha-linolenic acid include: purslane and walnuts; the Japanese use canola and soybean oils. You need a low-saturated fat, low-cholesterol diet; therefore, choose foods known to have low saturated fat and moderate to low cholesterol content. In this respect, the foods listed in Table 1 are recommended if a three-ounce portion contains less than five grams of saturated fat. The cholesterol content of most meats and poultry is similar and not excessive; therefore, no recommendations are based on the cholesterol content of these foods except for glandular meats, which are very high in cholesterol and must be avoided (see Table 1). Despite their high cholesterol content, eggs are an excellent and readily available source of nutrients. One egg can be used two or three times weekly, and at other times, an egg substitute can be used. A low-saturated fat diet has not been proven to decrease the risk of heart attack, but added alpha-linolenic acid to a low-saturated fat diet has proven effective in one study.

TABLE 3	List of Foods with Comparative Sodium (Na) Content	
FOOD	**PORTION**	**mg SODIUM**
Bacon back	1 slice	500
Bacon side (fried crisp)	1 slice	75
Beef (lean, cooked)	3 oz (90 g)	60
Bouillon	1 cube	900
Garlic powder	1 tsp (5 ml)	2
Garlic salt	1 tsp	2000
Ham cured	3 oz (90 g)	1000
Ham fresh cooked	3 oz	100
Ketchup	1 tbsp	150
Meat tenderized regular	1 tsp	2000
Meat tenderized low Na	1 tsp	2
Milk pudding instant whole	1 cup (250 ml)	1000
Olive green	1	100
Peanuts dry roasted	1 cup	1000
Peanuts dry roasted, unsalted	1 cup	10

The normal diet contains 1000 to 3000 mg sodium.
Daily requirement is less than 400 mg.

TABLE 3 cont'd	List of Foods with Comparative Sodium (Na) Content	
FOOD	PORTION	mg SODIUM
Pickle dill	Large (10 x 4 1/2 cm)	1900
Wieners	1 (50 g)	500
CANNED FOODS		
Carrots	4 oz	400
Carrots raw	4 oz	40
Corn whole kernel	1 cup	400
Corn frozen	1 cup	10
Corn beef cooked	4 oz	1000
Crab	3 oz	900
Peas cooked green	1 cup	5
Salmon salt added	3 oz	500
Salmon no salt added	3 oz	50
Sauerkraut	1 cup (250 ml)	1800
Shrimp	3 oz	2000
Soups (majority)	1 cup (250 ml)	1000
SALAD DRESSING		
Blue cheese	15 ml	160
French regular	15 ml	200
Italian	15 ml	110
Oil and vinegar	15 ml	1
Thousand Island	15 ml	90
FAST FOOD		
Chopped steak	1 portion	1000
Fried chicken	3-piece dinner	2000
Fish & chips	1 portion	1000
Hamburger	double	1000
Roast beef sandwich	1	1000
Pizza	1 medium	1000

The normal diet contains 1000 to 3000 mg sodium.
Daily requirement is less than 400 mg.

HEART FAILURE

Heart failure is present when the heart is unable to eject enough blood from its chambers to satisfy the needs of the body. Heart failure is responsible for over one million admissions to hospitals in North America. Heart failure is usually the result of a diseased heart. The commonest cause is a very weak heart muscle. The heart muscle is the strongest muscle in the body. During an average life span, the heart beats about 2.5 billion times, pumping more than 227 million liters of blood. If this work could be accomplished in one moment, it would be sufficient to lift a weight of about 400 million pounds off the ground. If the heart muscle is severely weakened and unable to adequately expel the blood brought to the left or right ventricle, blood backs up in the veins that drain into the left or right side of the heart.

Oxygenated blood flows from the lungs through veins to the left atrium and left ventricle (see Fig. 11). These veins in the lungs can become overdistended with blood and leak fluid (sodium and water) into the lung tissue. This is termed lung edema due to left heart failure. If heart failure continues for several days, the fluid may also accumulate in the space between the lungs and the chest wall and this is commonly termed water on the lungs.

The lung is like a sponge, and normally the spaces (air sacs, or alveoli) are dry and full of air. In heart failure, the excess fluid is in the spaces, as well as in the sponge work of the lungs. Thus, the lung is heavier; the fluid makes it stiffer with less capacity to distend with each breath; the individual therefore gets short of breath. The breathing is quicker and less deep than normal breathing. The fluid in the air sacs and sponge work of the lungs consists of water, sodium and some red blood cells. The patient may cough up sputum, which is sometimes blood-tinged. An individual with this type of condition is said to be in left heart failure or simply heart failure; because there is overdistension (congestion) of blood vessels and excess fluid in the sponge work of the lungs, the condition is also called congestive heart failure.

In heart failure, blood and fluid overdistend or congest the veins that bring blood into the failing muscular chambers; this congestion or visible distension of veins is seen in the lung on a chest X-ray.

STRUCTURE OF THE HEART

FIGURE 11

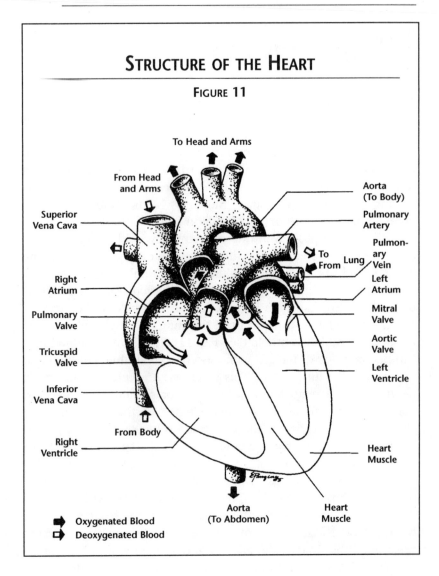

To Head and Arms

From Head and Arms

Aorta (To Body)

Superior Vena Cava

Pulmonary Artery

Pulmonary Vein

To / From Lung

Right Atrium

Left Atrium

Pulmonary Valve

Mitral Valve

Tricuspid Valve

Aortic Valve

Inferior Vena Cava

Left Ventricle

Right Ventricle

From Body

Heart Muscle

Aorta (To Abdomen)

Heart Muscle

➡ Oxygenated Blood
⇨ Deoxygenated Blood

In right heart failure, the distension and congestion occur in the veins of the neck, arms, liver and legs. The examining doctor therefore frequently looks for these distended veins (jugular veins) at the side of the neck which take blood from the head and neck into the right side of the heart (see Fig. 10). When a normal individual stands, sits or is propped up with the back and head elevated about 45 degrees, these neck veins are not visibly distended. In normal individuals they become distended temporarily when there is a marked increase in intrathoracic pressure as during singing, trumpet playing, coughing spells and the like. If these veins are distended and associated with shortness of breath, the doctor can be fairly certain that heart failure is present.

What about nonvisible veins in the body? The distension backs up in veins within the liver, which enlarges, and in some cases, fluid may accumulate in the abdominal cavity (ascites). The veins of the legs may not be visibly distended but the blood is under back pressure and fluid leaks out into tissues, especially when the individual stands, walks or sits for long periods. The swelling usually occurs more frequently at the end of the day, improves after a few hours in bed and is best in the morning. The fluid around the ankles and feet is commonly called edema and is a hallmark of heart failure, although it can occur with obstruction of the veins from other causes. This fluid is similar to that described in the lungs, consisting of water and sodium; therefore, the legs are brine-logged not just waterlogged. The swelling usually occurs in both legs whereas in obstruction of veins it is one-sided. The accumulation of several gallons of fluid may result in very extensive involvement of the entire legs, thighs, abdomen and lungs. Edema was referred to in the past century as dropsy.

Left heart failure is most often due to extensive damage to the muscle of the left ventricle as occurs during one or more heart attacks. Patients recover within a few days as the muscle is able to function well enough in the majority. About 30 in every 100 cases of heart failure persist in a mild to moderate degree, and medications are necessary. With the occurrence of several heart attacks, some being silent, further damage to the muscle occurs, leading to very poor heart function and heart failure. Such patients should not feel that it is the end of the line; many can live for several years provided that there is adequate medical treatment. Surgery is not usually indicated unless the muscle balloons to form what is called an aneurysm. Fortunately, this is rare, occurring in about one in 10,000 patients with several heart attacks. If the aneurysm can be removed, a reasonable cure is possible with major surgery.

Heart muscle diseases (cardiomyopathy) not due to atherosclerosis of the coronary arteries or valvular disease are fortunately very rare. In rare cases cardiomyopathy can be caused by alcohol abuse. Viruses that cause a very mild or moderate flu-like illness can cause microscopic scars in the heart muscle and weaken the muscle sufficiently to cause heart failure.

The heart muscle is commonly weakened over several years by high blood pressure. The left ventricle has more work to do to pump millions of liters of blood against greater resistance through tight, constricted arteries. The additional work causes the muscle of the left ventricle to increase in size much like the increased biceps of a blacksmith or weightlifter. The heart enlargement (cardiomegaly) is easily seen on an X-ray. After several years, the muscle is strained, and the patient may suddenly be stricken by an episode of severe shortness of breath due to failure of the muscle and a back-up of fluid in the lungs. Incidentally, heart failure appears to be precipitated in blacks much more quickly than in whites at lower levels of blood pressure.

High blood pressure may be limited to the arteries in the lungs (pulmonary arteries), into which the blood from the right ventricle is ejected. Such a situation can occur in patients with severe emphysema in which many lung vessels are destroyed, thus increasing the resistance and blood pressure in the lung circulation. The right ventricle enlarges and finally fails, causing right heart failure.

Diseases of the heart valves, for example, the aortic valve, can impede the free flow of blood from the left ventricle into the aorta; this is called aortic stenosis. When the mitral valve between the left atrium and left ventricle is tight, obstructing the flow of blood (mitral stenosis), blood backs up in the lungs and a cough with severe shortness of breath can occur.

In addition to problems in the heart and high blood pressure, there are several factors, listed below, that precipitate heart failure when the muscle is severely weakened. These conditions must be avoided or treated.

Problems that can precipitate heart failure in patients with a weak heart muscle include:

1. Patient-physician problems:
  • Reduction or discontinuation of digoxin or diuretics. The doctor may reduce or discontinue digoxin or diuretics or the patient may stop taking the medications.
  • The patient may increase the intake of foods containing excess salt.
  • Increased physical exertion.

2. Increased cardiac work, imposed on the heart precipitated by:
  • A marked increase in blood pressure.
  • Abnormal heart rhythms; e.g., atrial fibrillation.
  • Pulmonary embolism (blood clot in the lung).
  • Infection; e.g., pneumonia, chest, urinary or others.
  • Thyrotoxicosis (overactive thyroid).

3. Progression or complications of the basic underlying heart disease:
- Acute heart attack, several heart attacks or aneurysm formation.
- Valvular heart disease causing increased stenosis or regurgitation.

4. Drugs that weaken heart muscle contraction and may precipitate heart failure:
- Antiarthritic (anti-inflammatory) agents including indomethacin, ibuprofen, piroxicam and phenylbutazone.
- Beta-blockers.
- Corticosteroids (cortisone, prednisone).
- Disopyramide.
- Calcium antagonists; verapamil and diltiazem.
- Stimulant drugs that increase blood pressure, e.g., adrenaline, amphetamine derivatives and some cough and cold remedies.
- Alcohol, acute excess (e.g., eight ounces of gin in a period of less than two hours causes cardiac depression).

PATHOPHYSIOLOGY

When heart failure is caused by any of the diseases or precipitating factors outlined above, the body defenses are called upon to assist. Nature always has counterploys. Heart failure causes less blood to be ejected from the ventricles. Instead of about five liters per minute being ejected at rest, the cardiac output can fall to less than two liters and not meet the needs of the body. Compensatory responses of the body are the following:

- The nervous system and adrenal glands are stimulated to produce adrenaline and noradrenaline. Adrenaline constricts arteries and, therefore, increases the resistance in the arteries, which increases blood pressure to allow survival. This increase in resistance is a great load, which can be likened to a steep hill, against which the left ventricle must pump. The muscle is already very weak, and the increased workload increases heart failure. Imagine a 1934 poorly tuned car trying to climb a long, steep hill. Nature's compensatory responses are usually useful to the body, but in this case, they are counterproductive. The only way the heart muscle can do the work is to increase the contraction of the muscle and to reduce the resistance in the arteries. Nature unfortunately does not have a built-in answer and increases the resistance in arteries in order to increase blood pressure. The body is programmed to increase blood pressure when the cardiac output and blood pressure fall for any reason. Fortunately, medical scientists, by unraveling these mechanisms, were able to produce a series of drugs in the early 1980s that can reduce the resistance. These drugs are called vasodilators (see Heart Failure Drug Treatment).

- Two enzymes, renin and angiotensin, are activated. Angiotensin causes severe constriction of arteries and increases blood pressure. Renin stimulates the adrenal glands to secrete a hormone, aldosterone, which causes sodium and water to return to the blood vessels with the hope that blood supply and blood pressure will increase. The increased sodium and water returned to the blood by the kidney further increases leg and lung edema. Therefore, the body is once more deceived.

- The kidneys react immediately and utilize special mechanisms that cause a considerable amount of sodium and water to be returned to the blood vessels. The extra sodium and water again leak out of the blood vessels into the lungs and legs; thus, congestion and shortness of breath increase. You can understand, therefore, why doctors give diuretics, which cause the kidneys to excrete the excess salt and water, and this relieves shortness of breath and leg swelling.

As mentioned earlier, adrenaline is secreted during heart failure and causes blood pressure to increase and the heart muscle to pump more forcefully. This compensatory response is helpful and in some cases bed rest and oxygen with this normal response may cause some relief. Drugs, such as adrenaline, that increase the force of contraction of the heart muscle are called inotropic drugs. The best-known example of an inotropic drug is digitalis, which has been used for the past 200 years for the treatment of heart failure. You will note that the central cause is a low cardiac output, which seems to trigger the compensatory responses mentioned. Nature increases the blood pressure and heart rate but fails to increase the cardiac output adequately. It is blood pressure that is vital for existence. No blood pressure means no circulation to the brain and coronary arteries and, therefore, death. Researchers have endeavored to produce drugs that could increase the cardiac output when given orally without producing serious side effects.

DRUG TREATMENT

Digitalis (Digoxin)

In 1775, William Withering, a Birmingham physician, learned of a midwife whose herbal brew had cured several people suffering from severe swelling of the legs and shortness of breath. The condition at that time was called dropsy. Withering studied the brew and concluded that the only active constituent of the 20 or more herbs was derived from the foxglove plant (*Digitalis purpurea*). He used the herb with a fair amount of success.

Digitalis has been used extensively across the world to treat millions of people with heart failure. The drug causes the heart muscle to contract more forcefully and increases the flow of blood to the kidneys. Congestion, shortness of breath and edema improve. The drug also slows the heart rate and causes the heart muscle to use oxygen more efficiently. In some individuals, heart failure is precipitated by a very irregular heart rhythm called atrial fibrillation, and heart rate may increase to 120 to 200 beats per minute. In such patients, digitalis is very successful in reducing the heart rate to 60 to 90 per minute and causes complete clearing of heart failure. Digitalis remains *the only available oral drug* to treat heart failure caused by atrial fibrillation, and today this is its main indication.

Digitalis is not used in all cases of heart failure where the heart rhythm is normal, since in some of these, a diuretic and an ACE inhibitor bring relief.

Digitalis is available under various names. The most known and generally used preparation is digoxin. Digoxin is the purest preparation of digitalis and gives reliable blood levels. Thus, we will confine most of the remarks to this preparation. Other preparations have very minor differences in absorption from the gut, blood levels and duration of action. Digoxin is marketed under different brand names; *Lanoxin brand* is commonly used.

Supplied: Tablets: 0.125 mg, 0.25 mg.
Dosage: For maintenance, 0.25 mg daily usually at bedtime. In patients over age 70, 0.125 mg daily is usually sufficient.

As outlined earlier, digoxin causes an increase in the force of contraction of the heart muscle and slows the heart rate, especially in patients who have atrial fibrillation. The drug is excreted virtually unchanged by the kidney. Therefore, in kidney dysfunction or failure, the drug accumulates and can reach toxic levels in the body. Patients with poor kidney function may therefore require 0.125 mg daily or every other day.

Advice and Adverse Effects
Kidney dysfunction or failure is the commonest reason why toxicity occurs. Note that individuals over age 70 may have kidney blood tests (for creatinine) that are recorded as normal when the kidney function is abnormal. The doctor therefore has to titrate the dose carefully in the elderly to avoid toxicity.

Nausea and vomiting are common symptoms of excess digoxin in the blood. Blue-green-yellow vision may occur but reverts to normal as soon as the drug is stopped. Very slow heart rate, less than 48 per minute, with extra heartbeats and the precipitation of abnormal heart rhythms, is common with toxic doses. If this occurs, the drug must be discontinued and levels in the blood measured. Low blood potassium increases all adverse effects, and this may occur even with a small dose of digoxin. The potassium level in the blood should be checked every four months or more frequently in some cases. Diuretics are well known to cause potassium loss, and since they are virtually always used along with digoxin to treat heart failure, digoxin toxicity may occur, resulting in serious heart rhythm disturbances. Your physician will give advice on your diet, and tablets or a liquid containing potassium is required. Digoxin toxicity was common during the 1970s. We must emphasize that experts who have used this drug for over 20 years in patients with moderate to severe heart failure due to poor left ventricular function recognize clearly that when the drug is discontinued or the dose reduced, heart failure often recurs. We concur with this observation. Toxicity does not occur if the patient and a careful physician cooperate to prevent this.

Digitoxin

Supplied: Tablets: 0.1, 0.15 and 0.2 mg.
Dosage: Initial and maintenance doses are the same: 0.05, 0.1 mg daily; maximum 0.15 mg daily; digitoxin has a prolonged action and the effects can last four to six days. It is broken down in the

liver and excreted in the gut. Omission of a dose or kidney failure has little effect on serum levels. Levels are not usually increased in patients with severe liver dysfunction. The main "disadvantage" is that when digitoxin toxicity occurs, it can persist for several days.

ACE Inhibitors

The angiotensin-converting enzyme (ACE) inhibitors are very useful in the management of all grades of heart failure and represent a major medical breakthrough. They are considered vasodilators and have been shown to save lives and prevent hospitalizations.

Actions of captopril, enalapril and lisinopril

As outlined earlier, in heart failure the body tries to maintain blood pressure at all cost in order to satisfy the needs of the brain and organs. If the blood pressure falls, or the volume of blood reaching the kidneys falls, as occurs during bleeding or heart failure, the renin-angiotensin enzyme system is activated, and angiotensin is produced. Angiotensin is a powerful constrictor of arteries and increases blood pressure; but this increases the work of the heart and worsens heart failure. Captopril and enalapril block a "converting enzyme" that converts angiotensin to its active component. This new group of vasodilators are therefore called angiotensin-converting enzyme (ACE) inhibitors. The drugs cause dilatation of the arteries, reducing blood pressure and heart work. In addition, these drugs cause the kidneys to return less sodium and water to the blood, further reducing the work of the heart. The drugs conserve potassium, and as mentioned, a normal potassium level is essential for the prevention of digitalis toxicity and the maintenance of the electrical stability of the heart.

Captopril (Capoten)

Supplied: Tablets: 12.5, 25, 50 and 100 mg.
Dosage: Withdraw diuretics and other antihypertensives for 12 hours, then give a test dose of 6.5 mg daily, increasing to 12.5 mg twice or three times daily, preferably one hour before meals.

The maximum suggested daily dose for heart failure is 75 to 100 mg. The drug is excreted by the kidneys. If kidney failure is present, the dose interval is increased; for example, 25 mg three times daily can be reduced to 25 mg twice daily or to 12.5 mg twice daily. To re-emphasize: in kidney failure less drug is needed at longer intervals.

Advice and Adverse Effects
ACE inhibitors are not advisable in patients with severe anemia or severe renal failure. Do not combine with potassium in any form or with water pills that retain potassium. Captopril may cause a dry cough and severe itching of the skin. Increased protein in the urine and reduction in white blood cells may occur.

Enalapril (Vasotec)

Supplied: Tablets: 2.5 mg, 5 mg, 10 mg.
Dosage: 5 mg once or twice daily up to 20 mg daily.

Enalapril is an ACE inhibitor, and its effects are similar to those of captopril, as outlined above.

Other vasodilators used in the management of heart failure include hydralazine and prazosin, but their effects are variable and only rarely helpful. They are not ACE inhibitors and we do not recommend their use in heart failure except when ACE inhibitors are contraindicated.

Lisinopril (Zestril, Prinivil)

Supplied: Tablets: 5 mg, 10 mg, 20 mg.
Dosage: 2.5 mg once daily increasing as needed to maintenance of 5 to 20 mg daily.

Diuretics

Diuretics are a very useful category of heart medication. They play a vital role in the treatment of patients with heart failure or hypertension. In heart failure, the legs and lungs become not just water-logged, but brine-logged. Water in the legs, feet and lungs can only be relieved by using a diuretic, which forces salt and water from the blood into the urine. Severe shortness of breath and a feeling of suffocation is rapidly relieved by the diuretic furosemide. Diuretics used in conjunction with ACE inhibitors and digoxin prolong life and cause relief of symptoms.

Furosemide (Lasix)

Supplied: Tablets: 20 mg, 40 mg, 80 mg.
Dosage: 40 to 120 mg daily, for patients with severe congestive heart failure. Long-term maintenance for patients no longer in heart failure is 40 to 80 mg daily.

Nitrates

These preparations (see Angina) have a small role in patients who are not controlled with the use of digoxin and water pills, plus an ACE inhibitor. Their main action is to dilate veins, pooling blood in the lower part of the body. Less blood returns to the heart, and congestion in the lungs may be slightly reduced. This effect is only a mild one, however, and the drugs lose effectiveness if used continuously over a few weeks. They are often used in emergencies, in hospitals or, occasionally, at home to help patients with very severe heart failure get over a crisis.

Oral isosorbide dinitrate and other oral nitrates have a role; the preparation may be added to digoxin and diuretics and even to the vasodilators mentioned. *Some patients may feel dizzy*, however, with drug combination and close supervision by a physician is advisable to achieve the best effects.

Nondrug Therapy

Advice on Drugs, Salt, Diet, Potassium, Alcohol and Exercise

1. Medications must be continued as directed by your doctor. Do not stop any medications without consulting your doctor. Digoxin is usually necessary for a lifetime and diuretics for months to years and, in some, a small dose for a lifetime. We strongly advise you to take your medications with you on each visit to your doctor so that they can be rechecked or altered.
2. It is essential that you learn to live with a low-sodium diet. This does not mean that you must go to extremes and follow a 0.5 or 1 gm sodium diet.

   To achieve a low salt intake, consult Table 3 and simply do the following:

• Do not add salt in cooking or at the table. If taste is a problem, use a salt substitute after testing several preparations on the market. Salt substitutes have potassium instead of sodium and are therefore better for you but should not be used if you are taking an ACE inhibitor.

• If you have kidney trouble, you retain enough potassium; therefore, extra potassium not required. It is such an important and confusing area that both patient and physician must be careful. If you are taking an ACE inhibitor (captopril, enalapril), Aldactone, Aldactazide, Dyazide, triamterene or Moduretic (Moduret), do not use excessive amounts of salt substitute, eat a potassium-rich diet or take potassium supplements without the advice of your doctor. Appropriate advice from your doctor depends on blood tests to evaluate kidney function and electrolytes, which include blood potassium.

• Use foods containing small quantities of sodium. See Table 3 for sodium content of various foods. For further information on salt intake, see section in Hypertension (Sodium Restriction).

3. Apart from a low-sodium intake and an increased intake of potassium where necessary, the diet can be normal. There is no need to restrict cholesterol, fats or sugars since this adds to the patient's misery for little return. Such strict diets may rob the patient of one beauty of life, that is, to be able to enjoy a meal. This can result in a feeling of hopelessness and depression. Diabetics, however, still need to maintain their diets. Patients must lose excess weight to decrease the work of a failing heart. Less weight always causes less shortness of breath. A loss of 10 to 25 pounds always causes considerable improvement in shortness of breath and less medications are required.

4. The level of potassium in the blood must be kept within the upper normal range, 4 to 5 mEq/L. Except when kidney failure is present, extra potassium is often required in liquid or tablet form. The tablets or capsules may cause some gastrointestinal irritation. In addition, the pills are large in size and often rejected by patients, and they contain very little potassium. When a patient has a low blood potassium and kidney failure is absent, we strongly advise a potassium-rich diet because the liquid medications have such an unpleasant taste. Foods containing a liberal amount of potassium are given in Table 4.

The intake of foods listed can prevent the use of potassium pills or liquids. As an alternative, many doctors advise a diuretic that retains potassium such as Moduretic or Dyazide. In moderate to severe heart failure, a combination of furosemide, which causes a loss of potassium, and captopril or enalapril, which retains potassium, is advised. The various diuretics are discussed in Hypertension. Potassium chloride mixtures and tablets are given in Table 5. To be useful, the preparation must contain sufficient potassium with chloride.

5. Alcohol causes the heart muscle to pump less forcefully. Eight ounces of gin given to normal healthy students caused a 33 percent reduction in the amount of blood ejected from the heart. Can you imagine a sick heart with a handicap? If you have had heart failure, either do not drink alcohol at all or keep it under two ounces of alcohol, a pint of beer or two ounces of wine, on special occasions. Patients who have alcoholic heart muscle disease (alcoholic cardiomyopathy) should never drink alcohol.

6. Exercise or unaccustomed activity imposes increased work on a weak heart muscle and often precipitates heart failure. Walking is the safest and best exercise. Try to walk a half to one mile and stop and rest if you get short of breath. We do not recommend longer walks of two to five miles or jogging for patients with heart failure. Stooping and bending exercises may cause some dizziness, especially if you are on vasodilators, diuretics, and nitrates. Patients with heart failure, especially if recurrent, are not advised to engage in exercise programs even if they are claimed to be rehabilitation programs. Walking a half to one mile daily and stretch exercises should suffice. You can only strain the heart muscle; you could never improve it. We must re-emphasize that the heart failure that occurs during an acute heart attack is completely different and often clears within one week. Such patients can engage in various exercise programs.

WHAT TO EXPECT IN THE HOSPITAL AND ON DISCHARGE

The main symptom of heart failure is severe shortness of breath. Pain occurs only in those in whom heart failure is precipitated by a heart attack. If nitroglycerin is available, put one under the tongue and remain propped up in bed or sit until the ambulance arrives.

Oxygen is most useful and is given immediately. Morphine allays anxiety and pools blood in the lower part of the body; both actions bring relief. Nitroglycerin paste, ointment or patch is applied to the skin, and a powerful diuretic, furosemide, is given intravenously. Furosemide acts within minutes, pooling blood in the lower half of the body, and causes the kidneys to remove sodium and water from the blood and excrete them in the urine. Relief occurs within minutes, often before urine is passed. If relief is not obtained, further injections of furosemide are given.

The cause of heart failure and the precipitating factors are then treated, if possible. Fast, irregular heartbeat, atrial fibrillation, is successfully treated with digoxin. Hypertension can cause heart failure, and the blood pressure must be lowered. Preferably, captopril or enalapril is used to dilate arteries and lower blood pressure, and thus rest the heart. Patients with heart failure have a hospital stay of five to 10 days. Prognosis depends on the cause and precipitating factors outlined. Heart failure does not mean the end. Some patients do much less than before but they can live active lives for five to 15 years with good medical treatment. The reassuring news is that avoidance of precipitating factors can help enormously.

TABLE 4	Potassium-Rich Foods	
Orange juice	Half cup	6 mEq
Milk (skim-powdered)	Half cup	27 mEq
Milk (whole-powdered)	Half cup	20 mEq
Melon (honeydew)	Quarter	13 mEq
Banana	One	10 mEq
Tomato	One	6 mEq
Celery	One	5 mEq
Spinach	Half cup	8 mEq
Potato (baked)	Half	13 mEq
Beans	Half cup	10 mEq
Strawberries	Half cup	3 mEq
Avocado, meats and shellfish are rich in potassium.		

TABLE 5	Potassium Supplements		
Liquids	Ingredients	K+ mEq (mmol)	Cl- mEq (mmol)
Kay Ciel; Kay-Cee-L 1 mmol/L	KCl	20	20
Potassium chloride 10%	KCl	20	20
K-Lor (paquettes)	KCl	20	20
K-Lyte Cl	KCl	25	25
Kaochlor 10% (or sugar free)	KCl	20	20
Klorvess 10%	KCl	20	20
Kolyum	KCl	20	3*
Kaon Elixir	K gluconate	20	—*
Kaon-Cl 20%	KCl	40	40
K-Lyte (effervescent)	KH_2CO_3	25	—*
Potassium Triplex	not KCl	15	—*
Potassium Sandoz	KCl	12	8*
Rum K	KCl	20	20
Tablets/Capsules — Slow Release			
K-Long	KCl	6*	6
Kalium durules	KCl	10*	10
Kaon	K gluconate	5*	—
Leo K	KCl	8	8*
Micro K	KCl	8*	8
Nu-K	K	8	8*
Sando K	K	12	8*
Slow-K	KCl	8*	8*

*Note the low potassium and/or chloride content of some preparations.

Dosage: Usual range 20-60 mEq (mmol) potassium daily.

K+ = potassium.

Cl– = chloride.

HEART STRUCTURE AND FUNCTION

The human heart is a muscular pump. Its function is to pump blood containing oxygen, glucose, protein, fat and salts to every organ, tissue and living cell of the body. The heart is divided into four chambers (see Fig. 11). The upper chambers are called the right and left atrium, and the lower chambers are called the right and left ventricle.

Blood from all parts of the body drains into veins that empty into the right atrium. The blood passes from the right atrium through a valve and reaches the right ventricle. During contraction of the right ventricle, blood is pushed into the lungs, where it gives off carbon dioxide, takes up oxygen and returns via the pulmonary veins to the left atrium. During relaxation of the left ventricle, the blood passes from the left atrium through the mitral valve to reach the left ventricle. When the left ventricle contracts, simultaneously with the right, about 70 milliliters of blood are ejected with each heartbeat through the aortic valve into the aorta and circulated through the branches of the aorta that form the arterial system and supply blood to organs and tissues of the body.

If the heart beats 70 times per minute, it produces an output from the heart of approximately five liters of blood per minute; this is called the cardiac output. Each 70 milliliters of blood is propelled through approximately 100,000 kilometers of blood vessels. The heart beats about 2.5 billion times during an average life span, pumping more than 227 million liters of blood. Fortunately, the heart muscle is one of the strongest in the body. It can maintain efficient pumping and life for more than a hundred years provided that the coronary arteries that feed the muscle with blood do not become blocked by hardened plaques or a blood clot.

HEART TRANSPLANTS

Since Christiaan Barnard performed the first human heart transplant in 1967, success has been achieved in a substantial number of instances, encouraging enough to persuade various centers to engage in a heart transplant program. Despite recent break-throughs to combat the rejection process, this problem has not been conquered. There is hope that the results of massive research on the rejection process and its suppression will provide solid answers and most importantly drugs that will suppress rejec-tion without causing harm and suffering to patients. The next major drawback with any proposed heart transplant operation is the question of the donor's heart size. The transplant cannot be achieved if the donor's heart is too large for the recipient's heart cavity.

Apart from fighting the rejection process, the availability of human donor hearts of appropriate size and the question of AIDS will always present problems, thus limiting heart transplants to a few individuals.

HORMONES AND ESTROGENS

Normally menstruating women who are not on the birth control pill are protected from heart attacks. At age 37 the incidence of heart attack in men is 20 times that in women. Of 2,873 women who were followed for 24 years in the Framingham Study, no fatal or nonfatal heart attacks occurred in premenopausal women. Heart attacks occurred in postmenopausal women. The exact rea-son for this protection remains unknown and debatable. It would seem that a decrease in endogenous estrogens formed in the body increases the risks. It is difficult to explain why endogenous estrogens protect premenopausal women from coronary heart disease but not from the development of atherosclerosis of the cerebral vessels, which can result in strokes. In addition, in clini-cal trials on men who had a heart attack and were given estrogens, recurrent or fatal heart attacks were not prevented. The dose of estrogen used, however, was very high (2.5 to 5 mg daily), and cardiovascular death rates were higher in patients receiving the higher dose. Since it is known that high doses of estrogen predispose an individual to blood clotting, the results of that study are not surprising. The protection that may occur with the use of a small dose of conjugated estrogen (.3 mg) has not been tested.

Menopausal and postmenopausal treatment with low-dose estrogens (0.3 to 0.625 mg) decrease cardiovascular risk. If a progestin, however, which contains the female hormone progesterone, or its derivatives are added to conjugated estrogen, protection from the risk of stroke and heart attack is diminished.

A progestin is not required if you have had a hysterectomy. In patients who have not had a hysterectomy, a progestin is given to prevent the risk of uterine cancer.

Women perceive their risk of breast and uterine cancer as much greater than that of heart attack or stroke. Because of the increasing population of women over age 65 in the United States and Canada, cardiovascular disease causes a greater number of deaths in women than in men older than age 75. After age 65, one in three women has some form of cardiovascular disease.

Significant protection from heart attack and stroke in women can be achieved by the use of small-dose estrogen, e.g., .625 mg Premarin daily and 81 mg enteric coated aspirin (see Aspirin and Heart Disease). In some women, as little as .3 mg Premarin may cause a significant increase in HDL (good) cholesterol. It is important to increase the level of HDL cholesterol to give some protection from cardiovascular disease, which is expressed as heart attacks, stroke or death. It is difficult to increase the levels of good cholesterol in the blood by drugs, exercise or other means. New and expensive cholesterol-lowering drugs, such as lovastatin and simvastatin, do not increase good cholesterol. Women are, therefore, fortunate to be able to protect themselves before menopause; after menopause, they can obtain more protection than men from the risk of heart attack and stroke by the use of replacement small-dose estrogen therapy. In women with a predisposition to develop breast cancer, estrogen therapy is not advisable. The risk of developing breast cancer should be assessed.

The estrogen skin patch has not been used for a sufficiently long period of time to document its value in reducing cardiovascular risk. The estrogen in the skin patch bypasses the liver and may not increase the levels of good cholesterol; sound clinical studies to prove the value of transdermal hormone preparations are required.

Estrogens used as birth control pills cause a small increase in risk of thrombosis. The incidence of thrombosis in leg veins has diminished since the introduction of mini-dose birth control pills. The risk of thrombosis in leg veins and pulmonary embolism is still of concern in women who take the pill and smoke; those over age 35 are at high risk.

Birth control pills with fixed very-low-dose norethindrone, 0.5 mg daily or less, increase HDL cholesterol and decrease LDL cholesterol levels, which offers some cardioprotective benefits. Also, contraceptives containing desogestrel and norgestimate appear to have favorable effects on HDL and LDL cholesterol.

HYDROGENATED FATS

When liquid vegetable oils are chemically hydrogenated to produce margarine, *trans* isomers of naturally occurring *cis*-unsaturated fatty acids are produced. *Trans* isomers make up 6 to 9 percent of dietary fat intake.

The large Nurses Health Study in the United States showed a linear relation between *trans* fatty acid intake and the risk of coronary heart disease. Unfortunately, studies of this type use dietary questionnaires that yield biased estimates of intake. Individuals may report what they think they ought to be eating, or errors occur in recalling what they may have eaten five to 10 years earlier. A study in Europe and Israel (EURAMIC) in men after a heart attack, showed no effect of *trans* fatty acids on the risk of heart attack. Another study using the *trans* fatty acid content of fatty tissue taken from individuals does not support the hypothesis that *trans* fatty acids increase the risk of sudden death from heart attack. Further studies are required to clarify this issue.

HYPERTENSION

Hypertension, commonly known as high blood pressure, is a problem suffered by more than 60 million people in North America. The results of high blood pressure often lead to early death or serious physical handicaps. There are generally very few symptoms associated with high blood pressure. Dizziness and headaches may occur in some patients but generally health complaints may not surface for five to 20 years, thus the term "the silent killer."

Blood pressure is the pressure exerted by the blood against the inner walls of the blood vessels, especially the arteries. The blood pressure changes from minute to minute and is influenced by many factors such as activity, age, health, emotional tension and so on. With each heartbeat, about 70 milliliters of blood are ejected from the heart and propelled through approximately 100,000 kilometers of blood vessels. Constriction of the blood vessels (arteries) causes high blood pressure and greatly increases the work of the heart. Arteries are traumatized by high blood pressure and this increases the development of hardening of the arteries owing to plaques of atheroma (atherosclerosis). The heart may enlarge, arteries may become gradually blocked and circulation to the heart muscle, the brain and other organs may slowly become impaired until one day there will be an emergency situation such as a sudden heart attack or stroke. It is true that hypertension maims and kills millions through complications that are nearly all preventable.

Have your blood pressure checked. The onus is on you; you can save yourself from "the silent killer."

Clinical trials during the past 10 years have revolutionized the treatment of hypertension with and without drugs. Many familiar (old) drugs have been rendered obsolete because of safer and more effective alternatives.

If you have high blood pressure, safe and effective treatment is available either with nondrug programs or with a suitably selected drug. Drug selection is important and is discussed in some detail.

MEASUREMENT OF BLOOD PRESSURE

The instrument used to measure blood pressure is called a sphygmomanometer. It measures the air pressure needed to raise a column of mercury (Hg). The instrument consists of an inflatable cuff connected to a small bulb-pump and a pressure gauge. By means of the inflatable cuff, which encircles the limb (usually the upper arm), air pressure within the cuff is balanced against the pressure in the artery (usually the brachial artery at the elbow);

the pressure is estimated by means of a mercury or aneroid manometer. The mercury manometer is the most accurate pressure gauge. The aneroid gauge is frequently used instead of the mercury manometer since this is more compact and is convenient as a portable instrument, but it should be calibrated twice yearly. Some electronic instruments may give falsely high diastolic readings, but manufacturers will improve these to meet market demands.

The cuff size is of great importance. If the cuff is too small for the patient's arm, the blood pressure reading may be falsely high. In this case some moderately obese patients may be falsely classified as hypertensives if a normal cuff is used. A regular cuff may be used for arm circumference of less than 33 cm. A large cuff should be used whenever the mid-upper arm circumference exceeds 33 cm. The cuff must be applied snugly. To measure blood pressure, the cuff is wrapped around the arm about one inch above the elbow crease. Ask your doctor or nurse to show you how to take your own blood pressure. Occasionally both the radial pulse at the wrist and the brachial pulse at the elbow over which the stethoscope is placed are difficult to feel, and you may become frustrated with the attempt. Get your doctor to determine your systolic blood pressure using the stethoscope and also by palpation, i.e., using his fingers on the pulse at the wrist. Have him or her write down your blood pressure and you should keep this recording.

1. Remove restricted clothing from the arm to shoulder (no tight, rolled-up shirt sleeve).

2. You should be lying or sitting comfortably. The forearm should rest on a comfortable support such as a table at near heart level. If the arm is not well supported, muscle contractions will falsely elevate the blood pressure.

3. Apply the cuff so that the arrow or mark on the cuff is directly in line with the brachial artery (see Fig. 12). The arrow on the edge of the cuff is then approximately one inch above the point of application of the stethoscope.

4. Feel the radial pulse at the wrist. Close the valve of the instrument and hold the bulb in the right hand between the palm and fingers. Squeeze the bulb rapidly and fully. Continue squeezing the bulb several times to pump air into the cuff. The air pressure will at some point stop the blood flow through the brachial and radial arteries. Rapid inflation avoids trapping of blood in the veins of the forearm. As the

MEASUREMENT OF BLOOD PRESSURE

FIGURE 12

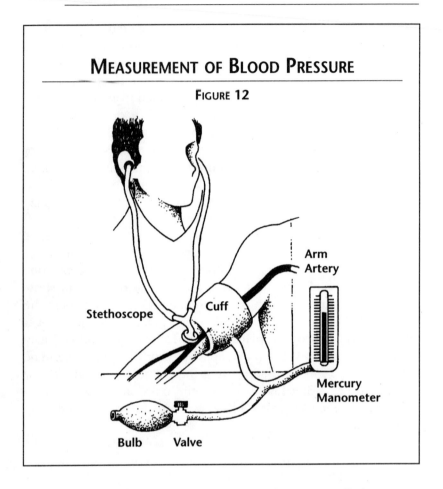

cuff is inflated the radial pulse at the wrist will disappear. Keep on pumping so that the manometer pressure is increased by another 20 to 30 mm Hg. Then gradually open the valve, decreasing the pressure slowly at a rate of about 2 mm per second until you can just feel the radial pulse. Note the reading in mm Hg. This is the systolic blood pressure by palpation.

To obtain your blood pressure using a stethoscope: If your systolic blood pressure is usually 140 mm Hg, pump the cuff up to a pressure on the gauge of 170, then put the stethoscope on the brachial artery (position as indicated in Figure 12), then slowly release the air. Suddenly you will hear thudding sounds, which are impossible to miss if the room is quiet and the stethoscope earpieces are fitting snugly. The sounds are produced by the blood being pushed by each heartbeat through the artery previously blocked by the air pressure. The air pressure recorded by the gauge in mm Hg at which you first hear the sounds is the systolic blood pressure. These thudding sounds produced by blood movement and vessel vibrations are called Korotkoffs sounds, as described by Dr. Nicolai Korotkoff over 70 years ago.

5. Further decrease the air pressure until all sounds just disappear and take the reading from the gauge as the diastolic blood pressure. Record, for example, as follows: "systolic 140, diastolic 80; or 140/80."

It is important to center the arrow on the cuff directly over the brachial artery. The stethoscope must be placed also directly over the artery. Your doctor can work out the line of the artery for you. The tendon of the biceps can be felt in the crook of the elbow and the artery is about one centimeter off-center, medial to the biceps tendon, i.e., nearer the body. Place the stethoscope in the crook of the elbow just to the inside of the middle of your forearm. It can be helpful to tape the stethoscope's diaphragm to the elbow if you are measuring your own blood pressure. If you wish to repeat the blood pressure reading, you must completely deflate the cuff and wait 60 seconds; otherwise congestion of blood in the veins of the arm can cause subsequent diastolic readings to be falsely high.

Occasionally it may be necessary to take blood pressure both in the lying and standing positions, especially if the patient is on medication. Some antihypertensive drugs cause the blood pressure to drop suddenly when the patient stands, and this is termed postural hypotension. In some patients over 65 years of age, markedly hardened vessels may require higher cuff pressures to stop the blood flow through the artery. This results in falsely high systolic pressure readings. This is one of the reasons why systolic hypertension in the elderly in the presence of a normal diastolic blood pressure is not often treated with drugs.

How High Is High?

The World Health Organization and many experts agree that in individuals under age 65, a systolic blood pressure above 140 and a diastolic blood pressure above 90 is abnormal. In patients age 65 to 80 a systolic pressure greater than 165 on three or more readings weeks or months apart is considered hypertension. The Framingham Study and other studies indicate a significant increase in cardiovascular risk in individuals with a blood pressure in the borderline range. An individual is considered to have high blood pressure if several readings exceed 140/90, especially if three consecutive readings are elevated. The risk at any level of hypertension, including borderline hypertension, is greatly increased by smoking or a high blood cholesterol. Mild hypertension is extremely common, and over a 10- to 15-year period increases the risk of stroke, heart attack and heart failure. Clinical studies have documented that blacks develop organ damage (stroke or heart failure) much quicker than whites at the same level of hypertension.

Your blood pressure changes from minute to minute and is lowest during sleep, dropping as much as 10 to 30 mm Hg. It rises in the morning and usually becomes higher in the afternoon. This makes it necessary to measure the blood pressure several times during the day and to record the time of the measurement. An average of at least three readings is often taken by the doctor. Blood pressure increases to the adult level by age 16. The systolic blood pressure tends to increase slightly after age 30. After age 65, a greater increase often occurs, owing primarily to hardening of the arteries, and a falsely elevated pressure may be recorded.

Hypertension is mild if the diastolic blood pressure is 91 to 100 or systolic pressure is 140 to 160. Hypertension is moderate if the diastolic is 100 to 110 or systolic greater than 180. Hypertension is severe if the diastolic is 115 to 130, regardless of the systolic pressure, and very severe if the diastolic is greater than 130 mm.

Prior to 1975, doctors believed that it was mainly the high diastolic blood pressure that was dangerous. An elevated systolic blood pressure, however, is as important as an elevated diastolic pressure. Such elevations in systolic blood pressure increase the risk of heart failure or stroke. The danger of heart failure is considerably increased if the patient has had a previous heart attack or heart failure, or has an enlarged heart.

The heart rate multiplied by the systolic blood pressure is termed the heart rate pressure product, and this product determines the oxygen requirement of the heart muscle. Elevation of the systolic blood pressure is just as bad as elevation of the diastolic in the range 95 to 110 mm. Elevation of either systolic or diastolic is important, but the combined elevation is more common and further increases the risks. Drugs that decrease both the blood pressure and the heart rate are more effective in decreasing the oxygen requirement of the heart muscle. Beta-blocking drugs play a very important role in the drug treatment of hypertension because of the aforementioned effects.

Over age 65, a systolic blood pressure greater than 165 is abnormally high; if the average of three consecutive readings taken over a period of weeks or months exceeds 165 mm, the diagnosis of hypertension is confirmed.

CAUSES

Primary (Essential) Hypertension

In the majority of cases of hypertension, no detectable underlying disease is present. There are several theories as to why the blood pressure may be increased. This type of hypertension is called primary to distinguish it from secondary hypertension, for which causes can be defined with certainty.

Primary hypertension has always been referred to as essential hypertension. The word "essential" was used because it was believed that higher pressures were needed to pump blood through arteries that were narrowed for some unknown reason. The use of the word has been so ingrained that it cannot be easily removed.

Secondary Hypertension

In only 5 to 10 percent of all hypertensive patients can an under-lying cause be defined. The most common causes include (1) kidney diseases, (2) coarctation of the aorta, (3) endocrine (hormonal) diseases and (4) birth control pills.

- Kidney diseases include infections such as pyelonephritis, nephritis (Bright's Disease), congenital cysts in the kidney (congenital polycystic kidney) and blockage of the artery that feeds the kidney with blood (renal artery stenosis). These conditions are easy to exclude by the physician's taking your history and examining the kidneys and urine and performing special X-rays such as an intravenous pyelogram (IVP) and arteriograms of the kidneys. The renal causes of hypertension occur in all age groups: children may get nephritis; blockage of the renal arteries may occur owing to thickening of the muscular wall of the artery, especially in young women; or in the elderly, blockage may be caused by atherosclerotic plaques.

- Coarctation of the aorta. This is a severe constriction of the large artery (aorta) that leaves the heart (see Fig. 11). Although present from birth, the condition may not cause symptoms and may go undetected into childhood or adult life. This condition is easy to exclude. The blood pressure is low in the legs and the pulses to the legs (femoral felt in the groin) are weak and delayed compared with the pulses in the upper limbs. Chest X-rays and arteriograms can confirm the diagnosis. In the majority of cases the condition is easily corrected by surgery. A recurrence of coarctation is success- fully treated with balloon dilatation (angioplasty). Long-term observation is necessary. The blood pressure becomes ele- vated temporarily following coarctation, then normalizes, but hypertension recurs years later in some. ACE inhibitors are preferred because the angiotensin system is stimulated (see Congenital Heart Disease).

- Endocrine (hormonal). This is usually due to an increase in hormone secretions from the adrenal glands. The adrenal glands lie on the upper pole of each kidney. The following are diseases of the adrenal glands:

    a. Cushing's Syndrome. Excess cortisone and its derivatives are secreted from the outer part (cortex) of the adrenal glands and cause hypertension. There is a redistribution of fat and a typical moon face, with obesity of the trunk; the arms and legs are relatively thin and the thigh muscles often become weak. Fortunately, surgery can produce a cure.

    b. Hyperaldosteronism, or Conn's Syndrome. This is due to a small benign tumor that secretes aldosterone. This hormone causes a retention of salt and water in the body and an excretion of potassium in the urine. Thus the serum potassium is low. The condition is rare and when diagnosed can be cured surgically.

    c. Pheochromocytoma. The center of the gland (medulla) produces adrenaline (epinephrine) and noradrenaline (norepinephrine). A tumor of this area causes excessive secretions and produces very severe hypertension. Fortunately, the condition is rare, about 0.1 percent of all hypertensives. The condition is important, however, since it is life-threatening, but when diagnosed, is surgically correctable. The features are often typical. In about 50 percent of cases, the blood pressure is relatively constant, and in the other 50 percent, the blood pressure fluctuates with paroxysms of severe hypertension occurring daily, weekly or monthly. The patient is quite well between episodes. During episodes symptoms include very severe, intolerable, throbbing headaches; profuse sweating and palpitations; fear of impending doom; seizure-like activity or psychoneurotic spells; weight loss; and postural hypotension (the blood pressure is very high, but may fall on standing). The blood pressure may be normal for several days or months and then suddenly rises to levels of 190 to 300 systolic and 100 to 160 diastolic. Fortunately, the condition is easy to exclude by urine test for adrenaline, noradrenaline, and breakdown products called vanillyl-mandelic acid (VMA) and metanephrines. A computerized tomographic scan (CT scan of the adrenals) will diagnose virtually all cases. However, doctors cannot run these tests on all of the 60 million hypertensives in North America. Therefore, the physician and patient should be alerted by such symptoms and initiate screening tests when warranted. Another important clue to the diagnosis is a failure to respond to the usual antihypertensive drugs or a marked increase in blood pressure that may be provoked by certain drugs. For example, the patient's blood pressure may increase with certain medications such as nasal decongestants containing adrenaline-like compounds, antihypertensive agents such as methyldopa and opiates such as morphine and Demerol.

Increased activity of the thyroid (hyperthyroidism, thyrotoxicosis) occasionally causes mild systolic hypertension.

- Birth control pills. Estrogen-containing oral contraceptive pills are an increasing cause of mild hypertension in young women. About 5 percent of users develop hypertension. The hypertension is usually mild, but rarely, severe hypertension can occur, resulting in kidney damage. On discontinuing the pill, the blood pressure returns to normal in the majority within six months. The increase in blood pressure described may be less with the newer low-dose estrogen contraceptive pill. The low-dose 0.625 mg conjugated estrogen used to treat postmenopausal hot flashes very rarely causes a mild increase in blood pressure.

MALIGNANT HYPERTENSION

This is a very serious condition. The diastolic blood pressure is usually greater than 130 for several hours or weeks. When such a diastolic blood pressure is associated with organ damage, notably to the vessels in the eyes, kidneys or brain, the diagnosis is confirmed. The blood pressure increases rapidly over days or weeks to dangerous levels, and the systolic may be as high as 250 to 300 and the diastolic 130 to 160. The retinas of the eyes often show hemorrhages and edema of the optic disc. Small arteries are severely damaged; in particular the kidney vessels are damaged and leak red blood cells. The urine therefore contains numerous red cells (microscopic hematuria). The function of the kidney rapidly deteriorates and a brain hemorrhage may also occur. Life is threatened by this severe damage to the kidney, brain, eyes and heart.

Fortunately, the condition is decreasing in incidence because of effective drug treatment of the moderate forms of hypertension. The reassuring news is that it is rare for a patient with the very common mild primary hypertension to develop malignant hypertension. The patient usually has moderate hypertension for a short period, blood pressure 200-250/105-120. In some cases the malignant phase is precipitated by kidney disease, such as nephritis, but rarely renal vascular hypertension (renal artery stenosis) or collagen disease such as scleroderma or pheochromocytoma. The malignant hypertension can be quickly brought under control by a range of effective drugs given intravenously. This form of hypertension cannot be treated without drugs. The blood pressure may be very high — 250/150 — yet headaches can be absent. Other causes of hypertension include brain tumors, bleeding around the surface of the brain from a ruptured artery (subarachnoid hemorrhage), spinal cord injuries and the well-known hypertension of pregnancy.

SALT HYPOTHESIS

The hypothesis accepted by the majority of researchers is that an inherited defect causes the kidney to retain excess sodium (salt) in the body. If you have such an inherited defect and your diet contains a large amount of sodium, your kidneys will retain more sodium and water. A normal kidney that has no defect in handling sodium will put out in the urine any excess that you may add in the diet. The sodium and water retained by the kidney get into the blood and also into the cells of the artery wall, thereby increasing the tone of the artery wall. This means that the artery becomes constricted or tightened and increases the resistance against which the heart must pump, i.e., there is an increase in total vascular resistance and an increase in blood pressure (see Fig. 13).

You may understand the relationship between salt and hypertension if you look at the following example: If an individual is bleeding severely from a large cut or from the stomach or other body site, the blood pressure always falls, sometimes to very low levels such as 75/50. A transfusion of blood must be given quickly to increase the blood pressure, because at such a low level, not enough oxygen, glucose and other nutrients will reach the brain, muscles of the heart and other tissues of the body. However, blood is not usually available in emergency rooms for a half hour to two hours. During this time the doctor rapidly gives sodium chloride (salt) diluted in water into a vein (intravenous saline), and this nearly always increases the blood pressure to safe levels until blood is available. During the bleeding described, the kidneys also immediately start to retain sodium and water and return it to the blood; i.e., the kidney gives us an immediate transfusion of saline. Nature always finds a way of healing!

Increased salt intake is believed to be the most important factor causing hypertension in susceptible individuals. The evidence is strong enough to warrant general education of the public. The U.S. Food and Drug Administration, the World Health Organization, the American Heart Association, the American Medical Association, the National Heart, Lung and Blood Institute, and two government-sponsored bodies in the United Kingdom have advised the general population to reduce sodium consumption where possible (see Table 6 — Sodium Content of Foods).

There is a considerable amount of scientific information that supports the view that increased salt intake causes hypertension in susceptible individuals:

- Population groups that consume very low amounts of sodium, less than two grams daily, have almost no primary hypertension; for example, groups in South America, Africa and the South Pacific. In contrast, in countries such as Japan

HYPOTHESIS FOR THE CAUSATION OF PRIMARY (ESSENTIAL) HYPERTENSION

FIGURE 13

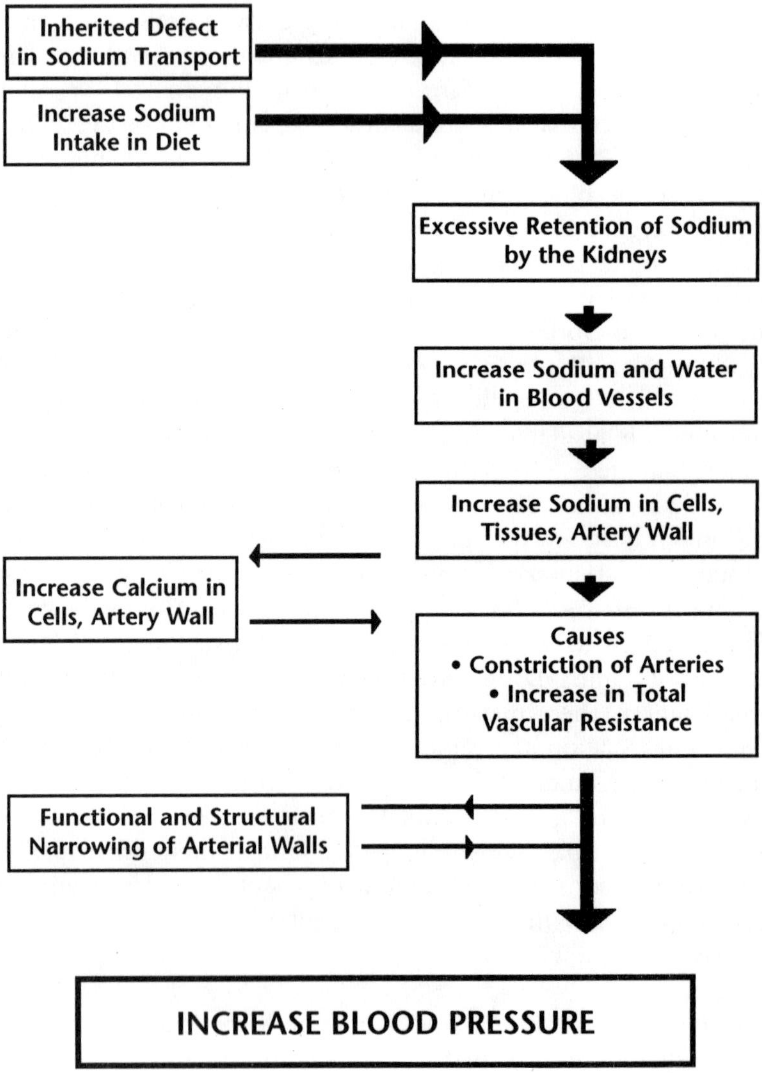

Inherited Defect in Sodium Transport

Increase Sodium Intake in Diet

Excessive Retention of Sodium by the Kidneys

Increase Sodium and Water in Blood Vessels

Increase Sodium in Cells, Tissues, Artery Wall

Increase Calcium in Cells, Artery Wall

Causes
• Constriction of Arteries
• Increase in Total Vascular Resistance

Functional and Structural Narrowing of Arterial Walls

INCREASE BLOOD PRESSURE

and Korea, where sodium intake is excessively high, i.e., greater than six grams daily, hypertension is very common.

- Twenty-seven studies in human populations have shown a close correlation between sodium intake and blood pressure.
- There has been a fall in the incidence of hypertension in Japan between 1971 and 1981, and this is believed to be due to a fall in the daily sodium consumption from above six grams to less than four grams.
- In Belgium, between 1968 and 1981, a fall in daily sodium consumption from greater than six grams to less than four grams was associated with a significant fall in mortality due to stroke.
- In children of hypertensive parents, increased sodium intake causes an increase in blood pressure and a greater rise in blood pressure after stress.
- Compounds that cause sodium and water retention by the kidney (hydrocortisone, licorice) often increase blood pressure. In patients with Addison's Disease, low blood pressure is always present and is treated with cortisone. Cortisone retains sodium with water, and this effect always increases blood pressure. Diuretic drugs cause the kidney to remove excess sodium from the blood and put the sodium and water out in the urine and thus cause a decrease in blood pressure.
- Patients with chronic kidney failure who lose excessive sodium in the urine tend to have a normal blood pressure, but in those who retain excessive sodium, blood pressure is often elevated.
- Animal experiments show a close relationship between salt intake and hypertension.

Despite the aforementioned points, incriminating an increased salt intake with hypertension, the Medical Research Council blood pressure unit in Glasgow headed by a panel of experts states that the evidence is unclear and unproven. Thus, they do not feel it justified to ask everyone to reduce sodium intake. We concur with this advice. There are many individuals who handle salt adequately. In this situation, we cannot advise everyone to reduce salt intake and we agree with the following: there is a consensus in North America and Europe that a moderate reduction in salt intake to less than two grams has no adverse health effects, and *whenever possible*, it would be prudent for the general population to reduce sodium intake, *in particular*, patients with primary hypertension and their relatives. If you have kidney disease, you should not reduce salt intake unless advised by a physician. (Some kidney patients can reduce intake.)

The evidence suggesting an inherited kidney defect stems from the work of Dr. Lewis Dahl, who bred two strains of rats, one that consistently developed hypertension when given an increased sodium diet, and the other that resisted the development of hypertension and never became hypertensive while on the same diet. Further, when a kidney is taken from a hypertensive rat and transplanted into a host rat with a blood pressure that is in the normal range (normotensive rat), the blood pressure of the host rat rises. A kidney transplanted from a normotensive rat lowers the blood pressure of a hypertensive host rat. It is believed that both the genetic and environmental factors (salt, stress, etc.) act together to cause hypertension.

OTHER HYPOTHESES

Other hypotheses for the causation of primary hypertension are shown in Figure 14. Hereditary factors and stress cause an increase in discharge from a center in the brain (sympathetic center), which triggers the secretion of adrenaline and noradrenaline. These compounds cause not only an increase in heart rate and cardiac output, but a marked constriction of arteries and increased total vascular resistance, thereby increasing blood pressure. This sympathetic stimulation activates enzymes in the kidney and adrenal glands (the renin-angiotensin-aldosterone system). Angiotensin is a powerful constrictor of arteries and thereby elevates blood pressure. Aldosterone, a hormone secreted by the adrenal glands, causes the kidney to retain sodium and water and this further increases blood pressure. The renin-angiotensin-aldosterone system appears, however, to have only a small role, and this is still undefined in the causation of primary essential hypertension. A low intake of calcium has been associated with an increase in blood pressure in two studies, but the evidence is not sufficient to implicate a low calcium intake in the causation of hypertension. Further studies are necessary to clarify the aforementioned theories of causation.

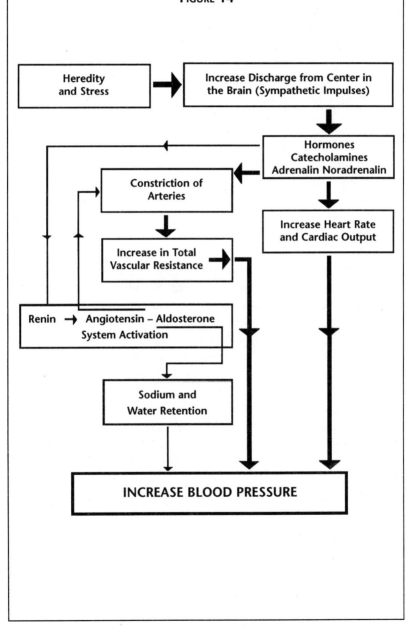

OTHER HYPOTHESES FOR THE CAUSATION OF PRIMARY HYPERTENSION

FIGURE 14

EFFECTS ON ARTERIES AND HEART

Hypertension damages the arteries in many vital organs, especially the brain, heart, kidneys and eyes. Damage to the walls of the arteries is due to the increase in blood pressure, but important added factors are an increase in pulsatile force and velocity of the blood. The artery wall responds to this stress by thickening its walls, but this leads to further narrowing of the arteries and a further increase in blood pressure. The arteries must branch to supply blood to various organs and tissues. Unfortunately, the branches to some areas take off at near right angles and mechanical stress is greatest at these points. The high velocity and pulsatile force of blood at a high pressure set up turbulence and mechanical stress that damage the smooth lining of the arteries, occasionally causing small tears (dissections) of the arteries. The mechanical injury provokes proliferation of smooth muscle cells of the artery walls and accumulation of fatty material including cholesterol and small blood particles (platelets). This thickening produces a plaque (atheroma) that juts out into the lumen of the artery thus obstructing blood flow, causing low flow and turbulence in the artery.

The term for hardening of the artery is sclerosis, hence the combination "atherosclerosis," meaning hardening of the arteries due to atheroma (see Atherosclerosis). This process is continuous over several years and produces no symptoms. On these plaques or damaged points, a blood clot (thrombosis) may eventually occur in vital organs such as the brain, heart or kidney. In the brain, a blockage (cerebral thrombosis) or rupture (hemorrhage) of an artery produces damage to a segment of cells, which results in weakness or paralysis of limbs and this is referred to as stroke. Each year about 500,000 North Americans suffer a stroke, and more than 200,000 die as a result.

In the heart, the coronary arteries feed the heart muscle with blood. A blockage of a coronary artery by atheromatous plaque or clot causes damage to the heart muscle, and this is called a heart attack.

High blood pressure causes enlargement and thickening of the heart muscle. These changes may be observed occasionally on examining the patient or detected on chest X-ray or electrocardiogram. At some point in time, the heart muscle weakens and thus fails to eject sufficient blood into the arteries to satisfy the needs of the tissues, and this is termed a failing heart or heart failure (see Heart Failure). Blood that cannot be ejected into the aorta backs up into the lungs, causing stiffness of the lung tissue and leakage of fluid into the air sacs (alveoli). These changes in the lungs cause severe shortness of breath. Heart failure can be precipitated by mild hypertension in patients who already have a damaged heart muscle, commonly due to an old heart attack (weakened scar). There are many other causes of a weakened heart muscle, however, hypertension of all grades is detrimental in all types of heart disease. In blacks, heart failure is precipitated at a lesser degree of hypertension than in whites.

In the kidney, hardening of the arteries leads to reduced blood flow and chronic deterioration of the kidney function, and this causes a further increase in blood pressure. Fortunately, only in patients with severe hypertension is kidney failure a final occurrence. The vessels in the back of the eyes may be damaged by high blood pressure, and the changes may be observed by your doctor if he or she examines your eyes with an ophthalmoscope.

Hypertension can weaken the wall of the aorta. The wall may balloon, and this is referred to as an aneurysm of the aorta. The weak spot may rupture. Rupture is often catastrophic and the condition can be confused with a severe heart attack; fortunately, this condition is rare (see aneurysm). The risk of narrowing or blockage of the arteries in the legs (peripheral vascular disease) is increased by hypertension, especially when there is either associated smoking, high cholesterol or diabetes.

SYMPTOMS

There is little doubt that hypertension either leads to early death or inflicts serious physical handicaps to millions. Blood pressure may be mildly or moderately elevated for several years without symptoms until the occurrence of stroke, heart attack or heart failure.

Symptoms may not occur for five to 20 years in the majority of patients with mild and moderate primary hypertension. Headaches, dizziness and nose bleeds occur with as equal frequency in hypertensives as in individuals with normal blood pressure. Some individuals get headaches during sudden elevations of blood pressure. Only in a few patients can symptoms be correlated with the height of blood pressure. Because your blood pressure may be very high and yet produce no symptoms, it is necessary to have a blood pressure check once a year or more often if you were ever informed that your blood pressure was above normal.

INVESTIGATIONS

Your doctor will very likely ask you to have blood, urine and other tests to determine if your hypertension is primary, i.e., without a cause, or secondary to diseases of organs, especially the kidney. The tests will also serve as a baseline for future comparison and as a means for detecting side effects of some antihypertensive drugs. The tests and the reasons for their use are as follows:

- A complete blood count determines the number of red and white blood cells in your blood. The red blood cells contain hemoglobin; heme is the iron in your blood, and this is combined with a protein called globin. The level of hemoglobin will indicate if you are low in blood (anemia). A very high hemoglobin (polycythemia) is a rare cause of hypertension.
- A test for electrolytes measures the amount of sodium, potassium and chloride in the blood. The potassium level in the blood is important as it may fall if you are taking a water pill (diuretic), which is commonly used to treat hypertension. The potassium level may increase with the use of ACE inhibitors.
- Either the blood urea nitrogen (BUN) or serum creatinine must be obtained. Urea and creatinine are waste products excreted by the kidney into the urine. The level of these substances in the blood is fairly constant when the kidney is functioning normally, but rises in kidney dysfunction. Your doctor will be able to tell from the results of these tests, as well as from urine tests, if the kidney is the likely cause of your hypertension.
- A urine test (urinalysis) may show excess proteins, bacteria or fragments of cells (casts) in the urine, indicating kidney disease.
- A chest X-ray is necessary and will tell the doctor if the heart is normal in size or already enlarged due to hypertension.
- An electrocardiogram can more accurately tell if the heart is enlarged and under strain. A chest X-ray cannot indicate whether the left ventricle of the heart is being strained by the high blood pressure. The ECG may also give other

important information. The reassuring news is that other tests are necessary in only a few hypertensive patients, perhaps five out of 100 patients.

- Intravenous pyelogram (IVP). In a few hypertensive patients with suspected kidney disease, this test may be requested by the doctor. A dye that can be seen easily on X-ray is injected into a vein in the arm and reaches the kidney within a few minutes. X-rays of the kidneys are taken over a 20-minute period. If the kidney is functioning normally, the dye is excreted into the urine and the X-ray will show the kidney structure as well as give some indication of kidney function.
- A renal nuclear scan may be done instead of IVP and is a safer test.
- Special urine tests for the breakdown products of adrenaline (VMA, metaphrines) as indicated earlier are rarely required to exclude a tumor (pheochromocytoma) of the inner part of the adrenal gland, which secretes adrenaline.
- A dye test showing the arteries of the kidney (arteriogram) may be required if your doctor suspects from the renal scan or IVP that the artery to the kidney is obstructed. This is a rare occurrence, about one in 1,500 patients.

NONDRUG TREATMENT

The majority of patients with mild primary hypertension are advised to persist with a one-year trial of nondrug treatment. It is important to understand the essential requirements of the program. The hypertensive must be aware of the dangers of the so-called silent killer so as to become sufficiently motivated to comply with self-imposed treatment. Individuals who persist with nondrug treatment have a 50 percent chance of lowering blood pressure to normal. The essential requirements are given in order of importance, and each will be discussed in detail below.

- Sodium in the diet should be reduced to less than two grams daily and at maximum three grams (see Table 6).
- Weight reduction is absolutely necessary and is always associated with a fall in blood pressure. The loss of 15 to 30 pounds always causes a considerable drop in blood pressure and medications may not be required.
- Removal of stress or learning to adjust to stress may result in

reduction of high blood pressure, and a trial of relaxation techniques can be useful in some individuals.

- Regular exercise will assist with weight reduction and relaxation.
- Alcohol intake should not exceed two ounces daily.
- The patient should reduce coffee intake and must stop smoking.

Sodium (Salt) Restriction

Sodium added at the table is only a minor part of the daily sodium consumption. A teaspoon, 5,000 milligrams of salt (sodium chloride), contains 2,000 milligrams of sodium (i.e., 40 percent). The body requires an intake of less than 400 milligrams daily. The daily North American diet contains about 4,000 to 6,000 milligrams sodium (two to three teaspoons of salt). Clearly no one adds more than a teaspoon of salt daily at the table or in cooking for a family. The remaining one to two teaspoons must come from the food we eat.

The aim is to cut sodium intake by 50 percent, to two grams daily. This can be accomplished only if the hypertensive or potential hypertensive recognizes and reduces or discontinues foods that have a high sodium content. The list is long and contains many surprises (see Table 6). The physician, the dietary adviser and the patient must be alert, checking the sodium content of foods consumed during one-week periods. Foods that are not salty to taste may have a very high sodium content. Note that some puddings have more sodium than a helping of bacon. A large dill pickle has more than one gram of sodium. Fast foods have a high sodium content (hamburgers one gram, three pieces of fried chicken two grams of sodium). Watch out for canned foods that have excess sodium added as preservatives.

Other high-sodium foods not listed in the table include soy sauce, onion salt, celery salt, seasoned salt, salted crackers, pretzels, rye rolls, salted popcorn, most canned vegetables, sausage, hot dogs, salt pork, sardines, smoked fish, TV dinners, buttermilk, waffles and pies.

It is obvious from Table 6 that the hypertensive individual must look at food labels and determine if foods have a low or high sodium content. Anything that has more than 500 mg per can is high. Additives are listed on tins in order of greatest quantity. *Sodium benzoate, sodium nitrate or monosodium glutamate means sodium.* Therefore, if any sodium compound is in the first five of the additives and the milligram content is not given, it is best to avoid the product. After a month or two of care, it will become second nature to purchase foods with a low sodium content. If you cannot avoid canned foods, rinse vegetables, tuna and the like under running water.

Low sodium intake is possible if you use fresh poultry, fish, beef, fruits and vegetables. Season foods with spices and herbs

TABLE 6	Sodium Content of Foods	
Food	Portion	Sodium, mg
Bacon back	1 slice	500
Bacon side (fried crisp)	1 slice	75
Beef (lean, cooked)	3 oz (90 g)	60
Bouillon	1 cube	900
Garlic powder	1 tsp (5 ml)	2
Garlic salt	1 tsp (5 ml)	2000
Ham, cured	3 oz (90 g)	1000
Ham, fresh cooked	3 oz (90 g)	100
Ketchup	1 tbsp (15 ml)	150
Meat tenderizer, regular	1 tsp (5 ml)	2000
Meat tenderizer, low-sodium	1 tsp (5 ml)	2
(Whole) milk pudding, instant	1 cup (250 ml)	1000
Olive, green	1	100
Peanuts, dry-roasted	1 cup (250 ml)	1000
Peanuts, dry-roasted, unsalted	1 cup (250 ml)	10
Pickle, dill	1 lrg (10 x 4 1/2 cm)	1900
Wieners	1 (50 g)	500
CANNED FOODS		
Carrots	4 oz (60 ml)	400
Carrots, raw	4 oz (60 ml)	40
Corn, whole kernel	1 cup (250 ml)	400
Corn, frozen	1 cup (250 ml)	10
Corned beef, cooked	4 oz (120 g)	1000
Crab	3 oz (90 g)	900
Peas, green	1 cup (250 ml)	5
Shrimp	3 oz (90 g)	2000
Salmon, salt added	3 oz (90 g)	500

TABLE 6 cont'd	**Sodium Content of Foods**	
Food	Portion	Sodium, mg
Salmon, no salt added	3 oz (90 g)	50
Soups (majority)	1 cup (250 ml)	1000
Sauerkraut	1 cup (250 ml)	1800
SALAD DRESSING		
Blue cheese	1 tbsp (15 ml)	160
French, regular	1 tbsp (15 ml)	200
Italian	1 tbsp (15 ml)	110
Oil and vinegar	1 tbsp (15 ml)	1
Thousand island	1 tbsp (15 ml)	90
FAST FOOD		
Chopped steak	1 portion	1000
Fish and chips	1 portion	1000
Fried chicken	3-piece dinner	2000
Hamburger	double	1000
Roast beef sandwich	1	1000
Pizza	1 medium	1000

Normal diet contains 1000 to 3000 mg sodium. Daily requirement is less than 400 mg.

instead of salt and use a low-sodium meat tenderizer. Onions and raw tomatoes can be used liberally in cooking. All hypertensives should have dietary counseling at least once yearly. The sodium content of several over-the-counter antacids, used for indigestion and stomach upsets, is high. There are, however, several brands on the market that have a very low sodium content, so please read the labels or ask your doctor.

Salt substitutes that contain potassium in place of sodium are helpful and can be used in place of table salt, except in patients who have kidney disease or take medications that retain potassium. You may need to try out several salt substitutes to find one that has a reasonable taste. Garlic powder but not garlic salt, onion powder but not onion salt, and chili powder may be useful to improve taste and yet remain low in sodium. Tomato juice and all the tomato sauces are high in sodium, but manufacturers are producing low-sodium tomato juices and a wide range of canned products.

Weight Reduction

A loss of weight always produces a fall in blood pressure and is therefore strongly recommended. Weight reduction has a greater blood pressure–lowering effect than exercise, relaxation techniques and or sodium restriction.

A weight-reducing, low-salt diet is often prescribed, but many patients fail to stick to a diet. Thus the diet must be individualized, and where physicians have little time to explain, it is best to refer to a dietary adviser, who can at least review the patient twice yearly.

Hypertension carries a greater risk of heart attack and stroke in patients with an elevated cholesterol. For patients under age 55, the serum cholesterol should be maintained at less than 200 mg/dL (5 mmol). The risks are considerably increased if the serum cholesterol is greater than 240 mg/dL (6 mmol). It is important when following a weight reduction diet not to increase intake of foods that are high in cholesterol. Low-cholesterol diets and the optimal levels of total serum cholesterol and high-density lipoprotein ("good") cholesterol are discussed under Cholesterol. Weight reduction diets must be individualized; therefore, no specific recipes are given in this book (see Obesity and Heart Disease).

Stress

The role of stress in high blood pressure is difficult to define. What is important is the way we handle stress. Stress itself rarely produces sustained hypertension, but in a susceptible individual with an inherited predisposition to hypertension, stress may increase blood pressure (see Fig. 14). It is important to recognize that an individual with an average blood pressure of 135/85, when under stress, can increase blood pressure 20 to 40 mm systolic and 5 to 10 mm diastolic. These increases in blood pressure may last minutes or several hours several times daily, and play an important role over several years. Thus, the patient with mild primary hypertension on nondrug therapy will increase blood pressure significantly during the day under the influence of stress.

The use of relaxation therapy has increased dramatically; many clinics offer facilities, although scientific studies have failed to show a sustained decrease in blood pressure due to therapy. On the other hand, studies are emerging that lend support to the salutary effect of relaxation therapy. Biofeedback-aided relaxation therapy seems to benefit some patients. This mode plus deep relaxation exercises are not harmful and can reduce blood pressure in some patients. Since the blood pressure tends to increase between periods of relaxation, do not rely solely on relaxation therapy if your blood pressure is greater than 160/100. Occasionally patients may need to change jobs or reduce workload, and to engage in hobbies, such as tennis, golf, swimming, fishing, painting, listening to music or other forms of recreation.

Exercise

Isometric (static) exercise, such as weightlifting (pulling, pushing), increase muscular tension and constrict blood vessels, thus increasing blood pressure. Such exercises must be avoided. Isotonic or aerobic exercises may cause a variable increase in blood pressure during the exercise and slight decrease immediately following the exercise. Walking, jogging, swimming and other forms of exercise should be encouraged in mild hypertensives. A fall in blood pressure may be related to weight loss and relaxation produced by exercise. If blood pressure remains elevated greater than 160/100 after six months of an exercise program, do not rely on exercise as a sole means to lower blood pressure (see Exercise and the Heart).

Alcohol

There is convincing evidence that any more than three ounces of liquor daily significantly increases blood pressure. Alcohol should therefore be restricted in all hypertensives. It is often stated that alcohol may produce relaxation, and two to four ounces daily may relax the nerves as well as increase the levels of HDL, the so-called good cholesterol. The risk of hypertension is greater than the possible benefits of a modest and variable increase in HDL cholesterol. If you have hypertension and previous heart failure, you should avoid alcohol. Four ounces of alcohol taken over a few hours causes a decrease in contraction of the heart muscle, thereby reducing the amount of blood ejected from the heart at each beat.

Coffee and Smoking

Coffee is also known to stimulate the sympathetic nervous system and can cause mild elevation of blood pressure in susceptible individuals, especially if more than three cups per day are consumed. Tea has much less caffeine than coffee and is not known to increase blood pressure.

Smoking definitely increases the cardiovascular risk in patients with hypertension. Also, *many drugs do not work efficiently* to lower blood pressure because *smoking interferes with their metabolism in the liver.* The patient must therefore be motivated to discontinue smoking cigarettes.

DRUG TREATMENT

Your physician will strive to use only one drug in the treatment of hypertension whenever possible. The ideal choice is a drug that is effective for 24 hours when given once daily, and that produces little or no adverse effects. Several drugs are effective only for six to eight hours and must be given two or three times daily. This is more cumbersome, sometimes more expensive, and often results in the patient's forgetting to take the medication, especially when the individual does not feel sick. Therefore, when possible, your doctor should choose a one-a-day drug for you. Occasionally the same drug is given twice daily and then once daily when the effective dose is achieved. This may not always be possible, however. A drug given twice daily may eventually prove best for you; therefore you must give your doctor the opportunity to manage your drug treatment.

There are more than 24 antihypertensive agents available. The doctor may state that the drug he or she is giving you is the best one for you. Yet on taking the drug, you may be the one to have side effects. Although side effects are fortunately uncommon and mild, you will need to discontinue the drug and try another. Your doctor should explain to you some of the problems associated with drug therapy so that you will accept and comply with drug changes, which are often necessary.

The standard approach to antihypertensive treatment is to use a beta-blocker or a diuretic as the initial drug. In recent years beta-blockers have partially replaced diuretics as the first-line drug, but both drugs are advocated by national consensus committees as the recommended agents to commence treatment except in special cases.

Experts vacillate between one drug and another as to their choice of a first-line drug. Other drugs can be used as first-line in selected individuals. Another important group of drugs that have proved beneficial in the treatment of moderate and severe hypertension are called ACE inhibitors because they block the action of a series of enzymes (angiotensin, renin). Angiotensin causes powerful constriction of arteries and therefore increases blood pressure when the body requires a boost in blood pressure. By blocking angiotensin these drugs cause dilation of the arteries and a fall in blood pressure. In addition they do not stimulate the heart to beat faster as do some drugs. They also retain potassium while diuretics cause a loss of potassium; this group of drugs (ACE inhibitors) includes captopril and enalapril. Another group of drugs recommended by the consensus panel are the calcium blockers (antagonists).

The drug treatment of hypertension must be individualized. In order to assist your doctor to accomplish this goal, you must give your past history of illnesses and your response or bad reaction to drugs.

- Your previous response or adverse effect to antihypertensive drugs should be a factor in determining further drug treatment.
- A beta-blocker (for example, metroprolol, propranolol or atenolol) is the drug of choice for you if you have angina or palpitations or have had a heart attack or have a strong family history of heart disease. Patients from 25 to 75 years of age usually respond to beta-blockers. Your doctor must respect the contraindications to the use of beta-blockers. In particular, he or she must not use beta-blockers if a patient has bronchial asthma or emphysema.
- Patients with stroke or poor circulation to the brain associated with postural hypotension (a big fall in blood pressure on standing), should avoid the use of methyldopa, prazosin or hydralazine and other drugs that cause considerable dilatation of the arteries on standing. Such drugs cause more blood to go down to the legs on standing and therefore steal blood from the brain, causing dizziness. It is important to note that beta-blockers do not cause postural hypotension and are therefore useful in this group.

Four main groups of drugs are in use:

- Beta-blockers
- Diuretics
- Vasodilators (including ACE inhibitors and calcium antagonists)
- Drugs that act centrally in the brain

Before we go on to briefly list the important drugs used in hypertension and some of their side effects and doses, it is wise to reflect on the following important question: *Is the choice of drug or dosage really important in reducing blood pressure?*

Consider the following points:

- It is not only the severity of hypertension that damages the arteries, but (a) the added pulsatile force of the blood; (b) the heart rate multiplied by the systolic blood pressure, which determines the workload of the heart and the amount of oxygen the heart muscle requires (thus an enlarged heart muscle working under strain will require more oxygen); and (c) the peak velocity of the blood multiplied by the heart rate, which reflects the turbulence of blood (turbulence causes damage to the inner lining of arteries). These three parameters can be favorably influenced by beta-blockers, made worse by diuretics or vasodilators such as prazosin, and not altered by drugs that act centrally in the brain.
- Beta-blockers are effective in preventing death in patients who have sustained a heart attack and are treated with these drugs for an additional two years. Four beta-blocking drugs have been studied in large clinical trials. Acebutolol, 400 mg daily, metaprolol, 120 to 200 mg, propenolol, 160 to 240 mg daily and timolol at a dose of 10 to 20 mg daily were effective in preventing fatal and nonfatal heart attacks. The interest should be centered on the potential complications, and not just the blood pressure. The patient is not only worried about his blood pressure but is afraid of stroke or heart attack. Doctors sometimes lose sight of this goal. They give drugs to reduce the blood pressure and lose sight of the fact that some drugs do prolong life more than others (see Beta-Blockers under Heart Attacks).

The answer to the question "Is the choice of drug or dosage important in reducing blood pressure?" is yes. The available evidence suggests that *beta-blockers have a definite advantage over diuretics and other agents as first-line therapy.* When utilized, diuretics should be given in the smallest dosage necessary to control blood pressure; i.e., hydrochlorothiazide, 25 mg daily. Hypokalemia (low serum potassium) must be avoided. A diuretic that conserves potassium such as Moduretic (Moduret) or Dyazide has a definite place in therapy if you have normal kidney function (see contraindications to Moduret or Dyazide use).

Beta-Blockers

See Tables 7 and 8 for dosage, and generic and trade names. Beta-blockers are excellent antihypertensive agents for the following reasons:

- They do not cause a fall in blood pressure on standing, unlike most other antihypertensive agents. Labetalol, which is really an alpha- and beta-blocker, does cause postural hypotension. This drug is useful in hypertensive emergencies, but we do not recommend it for the long-term treatment of hypertension because of potential adverse effects.
- The drugs produce no major side effects on heart, liver, kidney, blood or bone marrow.
- A one-a-day schedule makes it less likely for the patient to forget to take the drug.
- They can be used alone as first-line therapy and are effective in more than 60 percent of hypertensive patients aged 25 to 75, and used successfully in the majority of patients in combination with a small dose of a diuretic or with a vasodilator drug. They curb some adverse effects of vasodilator drugs.
- They prevent enlargement of the heart muscle, hypertrophy. They reduce the incidence of stroke, heart failure, heart attacks and deaths from heart attacks. Other antihypertensive agents only reduce the incidence of stroke and heart failure.

Commonly used beta-blockers include the following:

Propranolol (Inderal)

This beta-blocker has been in use since 1964, and is well known to most physicians. The drug is metabolized in the liver. It is strongly fat-soluble and therefore has a high concentration in the brain. This may be the reason for occasional weakness and fatigue, the very rare occurrence of depression, and vivid dreams. Forty-mg tablets are used twice daily and can be increased to 80 mg twice daily. Long-acting 80- or 160-mg capsules are available for once-daily use. Propranolol is the prototype of all the newer beta-blockers, and there are really only subtle differences. However, smoking decreases the effectiveness of the drug.

Acebutolol (Sectral, Monitan)

This beta-blocker has few side effects. It does not decrease HDL cholesterol levels or slow the pulse rate. A dosage of 200 to 400 mg once or twice daily is effective and is not altered by smoking.

Atenolol (Tenormin)

Atenolol is totally excreted by the kidney and, because of a long half-life, it is given as a one-a-day tablet. It is different from pro-pranolol and nadolol in that it is "cardioselective," i.e., it works mainly on the heart with only minimal effect on the lungs. Atenolol is therefore safer for patients with bronchitis provided that the dose is kept at a moderate level. If you have bronchitis, however, it is best to avoid beta-blockers. Atenolol as well as long-acting propranolol and nadolol have been shown to effectively reduce ambulatory blood pressure for up to 28 hours after the last dose. The effectiveness of atenolol, acebutolol and timolol are not modified by smoking. **Dosage:** 25 to 100 mg daily.

Metoprolol (Lopressor)

Metoprolol is similar to atenolol in that it is also cardioselective at low doses. It is a very popular beta-blocker and is used world-wide. This drug is given twice daily. Other features of the drug are similar to propranolol but there are fewer side effects. A long-acting tablet Toprol XL can be taken once daily and constitutes a major advance. Unfortunately Toprol XL is not available in Canada. **Dosage:** 50 to 200 mg daily.

Nadolol (Corgard)

Nadolol is similar to propranolol except that it is not metabolized in the liver and is excreted by the kidney. Because of its long half-life in the body, it is given as a one-a-day tablet. Insomnia and vivid dreams occur much less frequently with nadolol and atenolol compared with propranolol and metoprolol. If you get bad dreams with propranolol, therefore, we recommend switching to atenolol, acebutolol or timolol. The drug's effectiveness is not affected by smoking. **Dosage:** 20 to 120 mg daily.

Pindolol

Pindolol does not cause adverse changes in blood lipids as do some beta-blockers. The drug may not decrease blood pressure in hypertensives during sleep, however. The drug causes significant insomnia, disordered sleep patterns and in a few patients, nervousness, muscle cramps and joint pains.

Timolol

The drug is six times more potent than propranolol, so for a given dose, a better blood level is achieved with less variation. The drug must be taken as 5- or 10-mg tablets twice daily. Because of its potency and lack of anesthetic property, timolol is used as eye drops for the treatment of glaucoma. Smoking does not appear to decrease the drug's effectiveness.

Advice and Adverse Effects of Beta-Blockers

Beta-blockers should not be taken if you have chronic heart failure, bronchial asthma or severe allergic rhinitis. Circulation to the skin may be reduced and susceptible individuals may develop cold fingers. This is not a reason to discontinue a very useful drug. Remember the saying, "Cold hands, warm heart." Therefore, if you are really distressed by symptoms that can be due to any drug, you must discuss this with your doctor so that he or she can select another drug. The drugs produce slowing of the heart rate, but this is a desired effect and a reduction to 50 beats per minute is acceptable. Rarely the pulse may drop to less than 45 per minute, and if accompanied by dizziness and low blood pressure, the drug should be discontinued. Fortunately, the latter effect is uncommon, judging from the millions of individuals who are taking beta-blockers. Slowing of the pulse occurs to a lesser degree with acebutolol. The drugs may rarely cause fatigue, and very rarely mild depression. Reduction of libido and impotence are also fortunately rare. You must avoid stopping the drug suddenly. This withdrawal phenomenon is important only if the patient has angina or severe heart disease and is not important in patients with hypertension alone.

Beta-blockers reduce blood pressure and slow the heart rate. They reduce the work of the heart, therefore, preventing heart failure in virtually all hypertensives except the very few in whom the heart muscle is already severely weakened. A weak heart muscle may exist in patients who have had several heart attacks or who have severe heart valve problems. Such patients usually have low blood pressure because of the severity of heart disease. The aforementioned information, i.e., the patient's past history, makes it easy for the doctor to conclude that the heart muscle is weak, and this can be confirmed by the examination of the heart, the chest X-ray and the ECG. It is important to emphasize that large clinical trials of hypertensives utilizing beta-blockers do not show an increased incidence of heart failure. Clinical trials with timolol, propranolol and other beta-blockers in patients who have had heart attacks and were followed for two years showed that these drugs do not cause an increased incidence of heart failure. If patients are carefully selected by physicians, heart failure is not usually precipitated by beta-blockers and you therefore do not have to worry. Beta-blockers have been shown recently to benefit patients who have a mild or moderate degree of heart failure. This group of drugs is relatively safe and extremely important in the treatment of hypertension, angina and heart attacks.

Diuretics

There is no question about the efficacy of diuretics in mild to moderate hypertension, and when combined with other antihypertensive agents, they can be used in all types and degrees of hypertension. *The generic and trade names and maintenance dosage of diuretics are given in Table 9.* They eliminate salt and water from the body via the kidneys and are commonly called "water pills."

Hydrochlorothiazide

Hydrochlorothiazide is an example of a large group of commonly used diuretics called "thiazides."

Supplied: Tablets: 25 mg, 50 mg.
Dosage: Commence with 25 mg each morning and keep this dose as maintenance; maximum dose 50 mg daily.

The blood pressure–lowering effect is related to:

- A decrease in the blood volume. Patients who have an expansion of their blood volume especially due to sodium and water retention have the maximum benefit.
- Increased excretion of sodium and water by the kidney.
- Mild dilatation of arteries, thereby causing a decrease in total vascular resistance.

Contraindications:

- Hypersensitivity to thiazides or sulfonamides (sulfurs)
- Severe kidney failure
- Pregnant women and nursing mothers
- Patients taking lithium

A decrease in blood potassium does occur in a significant number of patients receiving thiazide and this is a potential danger. Diuretics also cause attacks of gout. The drugs cause an increase in blood levels of uric acid, and urate crystals precipitate in joints, causing sudden severe pain commonly in the joint of the big toe or ankle. The joint becomes very hot, red and swollen. Some individuals are very susceptible to small doses of diuretics and frequent attacks of gouty arthritis occur. Your doctor will prescribe a course of colchicine or indomethacin, and you will get relief in two to three days, then switch to another antihypertensive drug.

Some doctors add to the diuretics a drug called allopurinol to reduce the levels of uric acid, and this is given for several years. It makes more sense to stop the diuretics. The addition of allopurinol is a prime example of "poly-pharmacy," which adds to the handful of pills that patients are expected to take. It also adds to side effects and cost. We always advise patients to bring in all medications at each visit and these are reviewed. This verifies that the pharmacist released the drug prescribed. Drug interactions are a common cause of side effects that may elude physician and patient. We vividly recall the remarks of our professor in therapeutics (drug treatment), who made it a habit to remind us of the harmful effects of drugs. At least once weekly, his "Good morning" to the junior staff on the patients' ward would be followed by *"What harm have you done today, Doctor?"* His warnings have in some ways motivated us to write this book.

Furosemide (Lasix)

Furosemide is a powerful diuretic and is not recommended for hypertension except when associated with kidney failure; in this situation it is much more effective than thiazides.

Dyazide

Dyazide is a combination of 25 mg hydrochlorothiazide and 50 mg triamterene. The latter causes retention of potassium, and there is thus no need to take extra orange juice or foods with high potassium content. For dosage and side effects, see Moduretic. **Dosage:** One tablet or capsule daily. Larger doses should be avoided.

Moduretic (Moduret in Canada)

Moduretic is a potassium-retaining drug and contains 50 mg hydrochlorothiazide and 5 mg of the potassium retainer amiloride. **Dosage:** Half to one tablet or every second day, although the manufacturers recommend a dose of one to four tablets daily. Patients should not take more than one daily.

Dyazide and Moduretic are relatively safe when kidney function is normal; if kidney function is impaired such that the serum creatinine is greater than 1.3 mg/dL (115 μmol/L), these drugs may retain too much potassium. The two drugs are widely used in the management of hypertension and heart failure, and prevent the patient from having to take unpleasant tasting potassium chloride mixtures. Diuretics such as Dyazide that contain triamterene should be avoided in patients who are being treated for arthritis with indomethacin, and should not be given to patients who have had a renal stone. Moduretic and Dyazide should be avoided if you are diabetic and over age 65 or are taking an ACE inhibitor.

Vasodilators

By definition vasodilators dilate arteries.

ACE Inhibitors

ACE inhibitors are useful antihypertensive agents but careful patient selection is necessary prior to commencement of therapy. They prevent left ventricular enlargement, hypertrophy and heart failure and do not cause fatigue. Impotence is rare.

Captopril (Capoten)

Supplied: Tablets: 12.5, 25, 50, and 100 mg.
Dosage: 12.5 mg twice daily one hour before meals. If there is no major fall in blood pressure, the drug is increased to 25 mg three times daily to a maximum of 50 mg three times daily. A daily dose of 75 mg appears to be as effective as higher doses. It is advisable not to exceed 50 mg three times daily. If mild kidney failure is present, the drug is given only once or twice daily because it is excreted by the kidney and can be retained in excess in the body. These agents must not be used in patients with severe kidney failure, because too much potassium may be retained.

Captopril blocks the formation of an enzyme, angiotensin-converting enzyme (ACE), which normally converts angiotensin I to angiotensin II. Angiotensin II causes powerful constriction of arteries and increases blood pressure; when the enzyme (ACE) is blocked, blood pressure falls.

Advice and Adverse Effects
ACE inhibitors carry the rare risk of life-threatening angioedema that can produce swelling of the tongue and difficulty with breathing. Although this occurrence is rare, 0.2 percent of patients treated, the physician must warn the patient to seek assistance in the emergency room if there is swelling of the lips, eyelids or tongue. This reaction can occur within days and even up to two years from commencement of the medication. Deaths have occurred, albeit rarely. Mild hypertension is not a serious disease and many patients tolerate the effects for more than 30 years before developing complications. Thus, agents that are potentially harmful must be used only when other drugs are ineffective or not tolerated.

Captopril and other ACE inhibitors must not be taken along with potassium supplements or potassium-sparing diuretics such as Moduretic or Dyazide since they all cause a retention of potassium by the kidney. Cough is a common side effect of all ACE inhibitors. The drug rarely causes a reduction in white blood cells, loss of taste and itching.

Enalapril (Vasotec)

Dosage: 5 to 30 mg once daily.

The effect is similar to captopril; see table in Appendix A for other ACE inhibitors.

Calcium Antagonists/Calcium Blockers

These agents decrease the inflow of calcium into the muscle wall of arteries. A decrease in calcium within the muscle cell causes the muscle to relax, thereby producing dilatation of the artery and decrease in blood pressure. The level of calcium in the blood is not affected because the calcium is blocked only in the wall of the artery. Because these agents block channels in the cell wall that take calcium into the cell, they are also called calcium channel blockers.

Unlike other antihypertensive agents, calcium antagonists are effective in individuals at all ages and are even more effective in patients over age 65. Calcium antagonists do not cause life-threatening angioedema that is observed rarely with ACE inhibitors.

The calcium antagonist nifedipine (Adalat) has been widely used since 1982. Other calcium antagonists include diltiazem (Cardizem) and verapamil (Isoptin). Verapamil slows the pulse rate and should not be combined with a beta-blocker except in special situations.

Nifedipine (Adalat XL, Procardia XL)

Supplied: Tablets: 30, 60, 90 mg.
Dosage: One tablet taken once daily is sufficient to lower blood pressure over a 24-hour period. Usual dosage 30 mg once daily, if needed 60 mg, rarely 90 mg daily.

Adalat XL and Procardia are slow-release preparations that have proven superior to the older formulations, nifedipine capsules, which are used only in emergencies to rapidly reduce very high blood pressure.

This drug is very effective when combined with a beta-blocker. Thus a small dose of both drugs is often highly effective and has less adverse effects. Often physicians increase the dosage of a drug to levels that are advised by the manufacturer and adverse effects commonly occur. The combination of a small dose of two drugs is often better that a large dose of one.

Advice and Adverse Effects
Side effects include headaches, flushing, palpitations, dizziness and swelling of the feet in 5 to 10 percent of patients.

Diltiazem (Cardizem)

Supplied: Tablets: 30, 60 mg or Cardizem CD 120, 240, 300 mg.
Dosage: Cardizem CD 120 mg once daily increasing if needed to 240 mg, maximum 300 mg.

Advice and Adverse Effects
Adverse effects include mild flushing, rarely swelling of the feet, constipation and slowing of the pulse rate.

Verapamil (Isoptin)

Supplied: Tablets: Isoptin SR 120, 180, 240 mg.
Dosage: 120 mg daily increasing to 240 mg if needed.

Advice and Adverse Effects
Constipation occurs in approximately 15 percent of patients and is worse in the elderly. A slow pulse rate can occur.

Other Vasodilators

Hydralazine

Supplied: Tablets: 10, 25, 50 mg.
Dosage: 25 to 50 mg three times daily.

Advice and Adverse Effects
This drug was used extensively from 1960 to 1966, but fell from

popularity since 1968, mainly because it produced significant side effects such as:

1. An arthritis-like illness (systemic lupus erythematosus).
2. Dizziness.
3. Postural fall in blood pressure.
4. Palpitations (tachycardia) and precipitation of angina in patients with coronary heart disease.

The drug is relatively ineffective when used alone, although it is effective when combined with a diuretic and is more effective when a beta-blocker is added in a triple combination. The drug is contraindicated in angina and aneurysms. Oral therapy is recommended only when other regimens fail. The drug is useful for controlling excessively high blood pressure in pregnancy just prior to delivery. The drug is contraindicated in the first six months of pregnancy.

Prazosin

Supplied: Capsules: 0.5, 1, 2, and 5 mg (U.S.A.). Tablets: 1, 2, and 5 mg (U.K. and Canada).
Dosage: For mild hypertension, start with 0.5 mg test dose at bedtime. If there is no weak spell (syncope) or other adverse effects 12 hours later, then it is safe to take 0.5 to 1 mg twice daily for a week then progress to three times daily.

The average suggested maintenance dose is:

- Mild hypertension: 2 mg three times daily.
- Moderate hypertension: 5 mg three times daily.

A dose greater than 6 mg daily often causes an increase in heart rate and at this point the physician very often combines the drug with a beta-blocker, which decreases heart rate and further improves blood pressure control.

Prazosin blocks alpha-receptors in the walls of the arteries. Alpha-receptors in the artery wall, when stimulated, cause constriction of the artery. By blocking these receptors, prazosin causes the artery to dilate. The drug is thus a vasodilator.

Advice and Adverse Effects

An increase in heart rate is common, and while this may not be obvious to the patient, stimulation of the heart is perhaps not advisable. In this respect, the vasodilator drugs, by expanding the arteries, cause a fall in blood pressure similar to that of bleeding the patient. This produces a reflex stimulation of the heart and an increase in heart rate. With hydralazine, palpitations may occur in 25 percent of patients, and with prazosin, 5 percent; however, more than 20 percent of patients with either drug will have an increase in heart rate.

Drugs That Act Centrally in the Brain

Clonidine

Supplied: Tablets: 0.1, 0.2 mg.
Dosage: 0.1 mg at bedtime, and then increased to twice daily, with the larger dose at night. Maintenance dose 0.2 to 0.8 mg per day.

Impulses or discharges originate in the brain (sympathetic impulses) and reach the arteries and cause them to constrict, therefore elevating blood pressure. Clonidine prevents the discharges or impulses from leaving the brain.

Advice and Adverse Effects
The drug is contraindicated in patients with depression. Drowsiness is increased by alcohol and tranquilizers. Dryness of the mouth occurs commonly, and although dry eyes are not common, the patient still requires periodic eye examinations when taking this drug. Also, a severe increase in blood pressure (rebound hypertension) can occur if the drug is discontinued suddenly. We rarely recommend this drug.

Guanabenz

This drug has similar effects to clonidine.
Supplied: Tablets: 4, 8 mg.
Dosage: 4 mg at bedtime for one to seven days then 4 to 8 mg twice daily. A single bedtime dose is reported to be effective in some patients.

Methyldopa

Supplied: Tablets: 125, 250, and 500 mg.
Dosage: 250 mg twice daily increasing over days or weeks to 250

mg three times daily; 500 mg twice or three times daily.

It is postulated that the action of methyldopa is central in the brain, decreasing sympathetic impulse outflow.

Advice and Adverse Effects

The drug should rarely, if ever, be used without diuretics because it causes significant sodium and water retention. The drug is an effective antihypertensive agent when combined with a diuretic. Because of the potential side effects, the drug is now reserved for treatment of moderate and severe hypertension in combination with other agents when beta-blockers, diuretics or other drugs fail to achieve control. The drug has been used successfully for more than 25 years.

You should not take the drug if you have active liver disease or depression. The drug has been known to cause a mild hemolytic anemia, and so blood counts are necessary from time to time. If the drug is stopped suddenly, the blood pressure often increases over the next 12 hours to very high levels (rebound hypertension); therefore you must discontinue the drug gradually. If the dose is increased too rapidly, a sudden drop in blood pressure resulting in dizziness or a fainting spell may occur.

Other adverse effects include dizziness, sedation and sexual dysfunction.

Reserpine

Supplied: Tablets: 0.1, 0.25 mg.
Dosage: Initially, 0.25 mg once daily for two weeks, then reduce to 0.1 mg daily for maintenance. Maximum maintenance: 0.25 mg with a diuretic.

Advice and Adverse Effects

Contraindications include mental depression, active peptic ulcer, ulcerative colitis and Parkinson's Disease. If the daily dose is kept at 0.1 mg or a maximum of 0.25 mg, the side effects will be rare. Depression occurs in approximately 10 percent of patients with such doses; however, the drug must not be used if you have a history of depression. The drug has some advantages in that it is effective and economical and can be used once daily. The doctor does not have to increase the dose gradually over several months as is necessary with beta-blockers, prazosin or most antihypertensive agents. Reserpine in combination with diuretics or hydralazine is available in a single tablet and is recommended when other medications are contraindicated or fail to achieve reasonable control, or are unavailable. However, the reserpine-diuretic tablets commercially available provide far too much of each drug when the dose exceeds one tablet daily. Reserpine has been rarely used in North America or Europe since the late 1960s because of the advent of safer alternatives. The drug is of value and rightly used in countries where high cost and/or availability of drugs pose serious problems for patients.

Other drugs available for the treatment of hypertension are derivatives of the ones mentioned above.

Conclusion

Mild to moderate hypertension should be treated with one of the following:

- Beta-blockers, especially for patients younger than 75, and in all the patients with palpitations, evidence of coronary heart disease or those considered at high risk for cardiovascular events (angina, heart attacks, cardiac death).
- Thiazide diuretics in small doses, with special care to avoid hypokalemia (low blood potassium). From 1966 to 1984, the usual dose of a diuretic, such as hydrochlorothiazide, was 50 to 100 mg. This dose is now considered too large since it often causes a low blood potassium. The recommended dose is now 12.5 to 25 mg, maximum 50 mg. The use of a diuretic as the first drug to be prescribed (first-line) is particularly suited for patients in whom beta-blockers are contraindicated, and perhaps in blacks since it has been shown in some studies that diuretics are more effective than beta-blockers in blacks. A combination of one plus two is used only when one drug has been adequately tried, keeping in mind the risk of side effects associated with the increased dosage of a single drug.
- Other drugs are given a trial if beta-blockers and/or diuretics are contraindicated or produce adverse effects.

HYPERTENSION IN PREGNANCY

The safety of antihypertensive drugs is always a question in the minds of a doctor and, in particular, the pregnant patient. There are only a few relatively safe drugs available for use in the pregnant hypertensive patient. Thiazide diuretics are contraindicated because they cause a reduction in blood flow through the placenta and can produce a decrease in blood platelets in the fetus. After the first 16 weeks of pregnancy, obstetricians are satisfied with the use of methyldopa, but beta-blockers, in particular atenolol, have had favorable reports. If hypertension becomes severe during late pregnancy, the patient is usually admitted to the hospital and most obstetricians give a trial of intravenous hydralazine.

HYPERTENSION IN THE ELDERLY

Hypertension in the elderly (age over 65) is established when three consecutive blood pressure readings exceed 165/90. Often the increased systolic blood pressure is due to the hardening and reduced elasticity of the artery and therefore requires more cuff pressure to occlude the brachial artery.

The results of the systolic hypertension in the elderly program (SHEP) proved that the drug treatment of elderly patients age 65 to 80 with systolic pressure greater than 180 significantly decreases the risk of stroke and heart failure. The SHEP results indicate that it is advisable to treat all patients age 65 to 80 who have isolated systolic hypertension constantly greater than 180 regardless of the diastolic reading. A diuretic at low dose given once daily was very effective in the SHEP trial.

TABLE 7   Generic and Trade Names of Beta-Blockers

Generic	Pharmaceutical Trade Names
Acebutolol	Monitan, Sectral
Atenolol	Tenormin
Metoprolol	Lopressor, Betaloc, Seloken, Toprol XL
Nadolol	Corgard, Solgol
Pindolol	Visken
Propranolol	Inderal, Angilol, Apsolol, Berkolol
Timolol	Blocadren, Betim, Temserin

TABLE 8   Dosage of Commonly Used Beta-Blockers

Beta-Blocker	Daily Starting Dose, mg	Maintenance Dose, mg	Maximum Suggested Dose, mg
Acebutolol	100-400	200-600	1000
Atenolol	50	50-100	100
Metoprolol	50-100	100-300	400
Nadolol	40-80	80-160	160
Pindolol	7.5	10-15	15
Propranolol	60-120	80-240	240
Timolol	5-10	20-30	30

TABLE 9   Generic and Trade Names of Diuretics

Generic Name	Trade Name	Tablets, mg	Usual Maintenance, mg Daily
GROUP 1: THIAZIDES			
Hydrochlorothiazide	HydroDiuril, Hydrosaluric, Esidrix, Esidrex Oretic, Direma	25, 50, 100	25-50
Bendrofluazide	Aprinox, Berkozide, Centyl, Neo-Naclex	2.5, 5	2.5-5
Bendoflumethiazide	Naturetin	2.5, 5, 10	2.5-10
Benzthiazide	Aquatag, Exna, Hydrex	50	50-100
Cyclothiazide	Anhydron	2	2

TABLE 9 cont'd   Generic and Trade Names of Diuretics

Generic Name	Trade Name	Tablets, mg	Usual Maintenance, mg Daily
Hydroflumethiazide	Diucardin, Hydrenox, Saluron	50	50
Chlorthalidone	Hygroton	25, 50, 100	50
Methylclothiazide	Enduron, Aquatensin, Diutensen	5	2.5-5
Polythiazide	Renese, Nephril	1, 2, 4	2-4
Trichlormethiazide	Naqua, Metahydrin	2, 4	2-4
Cyclopenthiazide	Navidrex, Navidrix	0.5	0.5-1
Metolazone	Zaroxolyn, Metenix	2.5, 5, 10	2.5-5
Quinethazone	Aquamox, Hydromox	50	50-100
Indapamide	Lozide, Lozol	2.5	2.5

GROUP II: LOOP DIURETICS

Furosemide	Lasix, Dryptal,	20, 40, 80	40-80
Frusemide	Frusetic, Frusid	500	
Ethacrynic acid	Edecrin	25, 50	50-150
Bumetanide	Burinex, Bumex	0.5, 1, 5	1-2

GROUP III: POTASSIUM-SPARING DIURETICS

Spironolactone	Aldactone	25, 50 (UK), 100	50-100
Triamterene	Dyrenium, Dytac	50, 100	50-100
Amiloride	Midamor	5	5-10

GROUP IV: COMBINATION I AND III

Thiazide and potassium-sparing	Aldactazide, Dyazide, Moduretic (Moduret)		

Laser Therapy Versus Balloon Angioplasty

Currently many type of lasers are being tested. Lasers are capable of getting rid of plaques of atheroma in experimental animals.

In man, plaques of atheroma in the femoral artery in the thigh have been successfully dissolved by laser, resulting in relief of pain in the legs during walking. A few centers are doing experimental work using lasers to relieve coronary artery blockage. The laser is passed down a catheter to reach the obstruction in the coronary artery. The laser is fired, dissolves the blockage, and blood flow is restored to the previously blocked artery. Perforation of the artery is the major hazard. Unfortunately, recurrent blockage occurs within six months in approximately 30 percent of individuals. Laser therapy can be used when balloon angioplasty is not anticipated to relieve the blockage, for example, long or complete obstructions. A combination of laser and the balloon is used in specialized centers to clear blocked coronary arteries when the balloon alone is not suitable.

A combination of balloon angioplasty and a *stent* has been found to be an effective strategy with less tendency to blockage within six months. A combination of balloon, laser and stent is the next step. A stent consists of polished metal wires or tubes that are inserted into the artery after treatment with balloon angioplasty and act as a scaffold to maintain patency of the treated artery.

Murmurs

Murmurs are most commonly systolic in time; that is, they occur during the contraction of the ventricles. Many systolic murmurs are not significant in that they do not disturb the function of the heart. Murmurs that occur when the ventricles are relaxed, that is, during diastole, are termed diastolic murmurs and are always of significance. Murmurs are usually caused by disease of the heart valves (see Valve Diseases).

Over of a period of five to 50 years, significant murmurs increase the work of the heart muscle and cause it to enlarge. The muscle finally becomes weak and heart failure occurs. When heart failure occurs, it is not the end of the life (see Heart Failure).

QUESTIONS POSED

A female, age 30, posed the following questions: My family doctor says that I have a systolic murmur at the apex of the heart and referred me to a cardiologist. I would like to know:

1. What is my prognosis?
2. Is there any contraindication to using the birth control pill?
3. Will the murmur affect future pregnancy and the number of children I can have?
4. When will an operation be necessary?
5. Can I prevent it from becoming worse?

ANSWERS

1. A soft systolic murmur over the apex of the heart is usually of no significance. It is important, however, to identify any mild area of roughness or deformity of the valve, which can later develop an infection called endocarditis. When a doctor states that a murmur is of no significance, it means that the murmur will not affect the person's life span or activities. If you have not had rheumatic fever and there are no other murmurs and no shortness of breath, the murmur is likely due to an increased blood flow across the valve, a common finding in normal young adults and also during pregnancy. The cardiologist's findings with the stethoscope, followed by a chest X-ray and electrocardiogram, usually exclude most serious problems. If some doubt exists, an echocardiogram is helpful. Echocardiography will document a degree of stenosis, or regurgitation. Diastolic murmurs are always significant whereas soft systolic murmurs are often not of significance.
2. The murmur does not contraindicate the use of the birth control pill.
3. The murmur will not affect your pregnancy, the fetus or subsequent pregnancies and should not limit the number of

children. If the murmur is loud and the doctor hears it over a wide area of the chest, this is a different matter and further assessment including an echocardiogram may be necessary to exclude severe mitral regurgitation.

4. An operation is never required in patients with a soft systolic murmur or mild mitral regurgitation. Surgery for mitral regurgitation is utilized only when there are symptoms of severe shortness of breath or heart enlargement and when an echocardiogram shows severe regurgitation.

5. If you have no symptoms and if the murmur is described as soft and heard over an area of less than five fingertips held together, it is most unlikely that your condition will get worse. Only infection of the valve can shorten your life. Fortunately, the risk of getting an infection on the valve is remote; when germs get into the blood, they need to stick on the valve and grow. There is a one in 1,000 chance of this occurring, and prevention through antibiotics is the rule if the murmur is caused by a valve disease process. Antibiotics are not required for many "funtional," nonsignificant murmurs (see Dental Work and Heart Disease).

DIAGNOSIS OF HEART MURMUR AND TESTS REQUIRED

Usually the diagnosis is obvious from the patient's history of shortness of breath and the finding of a murmur with the stethoscope. A cardiologist makes the diagnosis in the office with 95 percent confidence in more than 95 percent of cases. The chest X-ray, ECG and echocardiogram are helpful to confirm the opinion. In a few individuals with serious heart murmurs causing symptoms such as severe shortness of breath with or without heart failure, catheter tests are invaluable and must be done if surgical correction is planned. The technique of catheterization is outlined under Tests for Heart Diseases.

Nonsteroidal Antiinflammatory Agents (NSAIDs)

These agents are widely used for the control of pain in patients with arthritis. NSAIDs cause the kidneys to retain sodium and water. This action may cause an increase in blood pressure. Also, an increase in sodium and water in the body increases the work of the heart and can precipitate heart failure. Patients may experience increased shortness of breath and swelling of the ankles. Available NSAIDs include carprofen, diclofenac, fenoprofen, flurbiprofen, ibuprofen, indomethacin, ketoprofen, naproxen, piroxicam, sulindac and tolmetin.

NSAIDs significantly inhibit the beneficial effects of several drugs, including those used to treat high blood pressure and heart failure, particularly, furosemide, hydrochlorothiazide and ACE inhibitors. Aspirin is a weak NSAID and fortunately does not cause sodium and water retention, increased blood pressure or heart failure, but it can interfere with the effectiveness of ACE inhibitors.

Obesity and Heart Disease

If you are slightly overweight, this does not increase your risk of having a heart attack, provided that you do not have other risk factors — especially hypertension, high blood cholesterol, smoking and diabetes.

The Metropolitan height and weight tables are given in Tables 10 and 11. If you are slightly overweight, you would be happy to learn that the earlier Metropolitan Life tables of ideal or average weights were derived from insurance applicants age 20 to 30 and do not represent the average weights of individuals age 40 to 60. If your weight is 10 percent more than that indicated in Table 10 or 11, you can consider yourself slightly overweight, but there is still no health hazard unless you have other risk factors. The average weight of North Americans age 30 to 50 is about 10 to 15 percent above those indicated in Tables 10 and 11. Many North Americans age 35 to 65 are overweight, even by the conservative definition given above. If you are in this group and have other risk factors, you need to reduce your weight. The Framingham Study showed that in the 5,000 people studied, being overweight appeared to increase the risk of sudden death and angina, but it did not increase the frequency of heart attacks. When adjustments were made for the prevalence of hypertension and hypercholesterolemia, then overweight or obesity appeared to play a much less significant role.

If a patient with chest pain due to coronary heart disease is overweight, chest pains are likely to be more frequent, as the heart certainly has more work to do. Therefore, weight reduction does help in relieving pain in patients with angina pectoris, and it is strongly advisable: less drugs are then required.

TABLE 10 1983 Metropolitan Life Height and Weight Tables for Men and Women According to Frame, Ages 25-59: Men

Height (in Shoes) Feet Inches	Weight in Pounds (in Indoor Clothing)*		
	Small Frame	Medium Frame	Large Frame
5 2	128-134	131-141	138-150
5 3	130-136	133-143	140-153
5 4	132-138	135-145	142-156
5 5	134-140	137-148	144-160
5 6	136-142	139-151	146-164
5 7	138-145	142-154	149-168
5 8	140-148	145-157	152-172
5 9	142-151	148-160	155-176
5 10	144-154	151-163	158-180
5 11	146-157	154-166	161-184
6 0	149-160	157-170	164-188
6 1	152-164	160-174	168-192
6 2	155-168	164-178	172-197
6 3	158-172	167-182	176-202
6 4	162-176	171-187	181-207

* Indoor clothing weighing 5 pounds for men and 3 pounds for women.

You are considered obese if you are more than 25 percent above the average weight and have a high percentage of body fat. You are moderately obese if you are 25 to 50 percent above the average weight and have marked increase in body fat. Measurement of body mass index, from your weight divided by the square of your height, is a useful measure of relative obesity.

Obesity is not a major cause of hypertension, but some obese patients do have an increase in blood pressure. A larger sized cuff is required for measuring blood pressure if the individual's arm is large. If you are obese and lose weight, the blood pressure always falls. A significant number of obese patients have diabetes and elevated blood cholesterol, and if hypertension or cigarette smoking is added, the risk is considerably increased.

TABLE 11 **1983 Metropolitan Life Height and Weight Tables for Men and Women According to Frame, Ages 25-59: Women**

Height (In Shoes) Feet Inches	Small Frame	Medium Frame	Large Frame
4 10	102-111	109-121	118-131
4 11	103-113	111-123	120-134
5 0	104-115	113-126	122-137
5 1	106-118	115-129	125-140
5 2	108-121	118-132	128-143
5 3	111-124	121-135	131-147
5 4	114-127	124-138	134-151
5 5	117-130	127-141	137-155
5 6	120-133	130-144	140-159
5 7	123-136	133-147	143-163
5 8	126-139	136-150	146-167
5 9	129-142	139-153	149-170
5 10	132-145	142-156	152-173
5 11	135-148	145-159	155-176
6 0	138-151	148-162	158-179

Weight in Pounds (in Indoor Clothing)*

*Shoes with 1-inch heels.

Source of basic data: *Build Study, 1979,* Society of Actuaries and Association of Life Insurance Medical Directors of America, 1980.

Copyright 1983 Metropolitan Life Insurance Company.

WEIGHT REDUCTION DIET

Weight loss depends on:

- calories you do not eat and
- calories you burn up during exercise.

A low-calorie diet must be combined with exercise that increases calorie expenditure; otherwise you will not be able to prevent weight gain, which often occurs three to six months after stopping a low-calorie diet. It is best to lose slowly and plan your strategy over a one-year period. Therefore, try to lose two to four pounds per month, that is, 24 to 48 pounds over one year.

The body of an obese individual is programmed to form fat and store it. In addition, cells slow down and you burn fewer calories than normal. Your metabolic rate is slower than normal. When you go on a crash diet, your metabolic thermostat is turned down to get by on less food. Start your exercise program first, and after a month of walking one to two miles daily and climbing two to three flights of stairs four times daily, increase the exercise and then start your diet. Remember that a brisk two-mile walk in 30 minutes burns about 200 calories.

All weight reduction diets entail a major reduction in simple carbohydrate foods (sugar and starchy foods), which break down in the body to form glucose (sugar). Therefore, you need to make a list of all such foods and reduce them by 50 to 75 percent (one half to three quarters) of your usual intake. We have not printed such a list, since they are readily available in most diet books. A decrease in saturated fat as advised in our Heart Attack Prevention Diet is advisable. Total fat intake should be reduced from the average 40 percent of total caloric intake to 30 percent. One gram of fat is equal to 9 calories, thus reducing fat intake by 120 calories derived from fat is not a difficult undertaking. A filet mignon is not fattening. Thus you can eat filet mignon and chicken three times a week and still lose weight.

All diets that are proven to cause sustained weight loss over a period of years depend on a reduced intake of calories. Therefore, calories do count. Don't let anyone tell you otherwise. Most calories are derived from carbohydrates: flour products, potatoes, ground vegetables, rice, custard, ice cream and the like. A smaller amount of calories are derived from lean meats. To lose weight, therefore, eat only vegetables and lean meats, chicken and fish; fruit for dessert.

Your cells and muscles need energy to carry out their work. Energy is measured in calories. The body cells are like light bulbs. A bulb lights up when it receives enough electrical energy. The cells derive energy from chemical reactions involving glucose, oxygen, hydrogen and high-energy phosphate bonds. The body needs glucose because it is one of the chief sources of energy — calories. The following example should help you understand weight loss and calories. Young diabetics lose a considerable amount of weight. Why? Insulin is required to transport glucose from the blood across the cell membrane to reach inside the cell to interact with other chemicals and so produce energy. When insulin is absent, glucose cannot get into the cells. Therefore, glucose reaches high levels in the blood and is passed out in the urine. The cells require energy to accomplish their particular function. When glucose is not present, the cells use fat as a source of energy. Thus, fat throughout the body is mobilized and broken down, resulting in marked weight loss, 20 to 30 pounds in two to three months.

Weight loss will be achieved if you reduce your calorie intake to 1,000 calories daily and burn up some calories by exercise. It is possible to eat attractive, appetizing meals and lose weight. Consider the following points in preparing your meals:

1. A meal containing high protein and low-to-moderate fat, as detailed under Heart Attack Prevention Diet, is advisable.
2. Reduce intake of high-calorie foods: carbohydrate consisting of refined sugars and refined starches. Remember that alcohol, mixes, beer and soft drinks contain an abundance of calories.
3. Carbohydrate foods that have calories and can still be taken liberally include those containing high fiber. Foods with high fiber content allow you to eat a large meal; therefore, you feel satisfied. Most of the material stays longer in the stomach but is not digested and thus not absorbed into the blood. Your meal may have more calories, but you absorb only about half the amount of calories. We agree that high-fiber diets have a definite role in weight reduction plans. High-fiber foods include: wheat bran, green peas, chick peas, split peas, beans, corn, all vegetables and fruits — in particular apples, pears, plums, nectarines and the like, since the skin containing high fiber is eaten.

We must issue a word of caution, however: Every intervention, be it type of diet or treatment, must be done in moderation. We must draw your attention to the high vitamin K content of certain high-fiber foods often recommended — broccoli, turnip greens, spinach and alfalfa. A high vitamin K intake may increase clotting factors in the blood. In addition, the occasional individual following a high-fiber diet may have an increase in stools from once to three times daily, but this often normalizes. Very rarely anemia and bone loss (osteomalacia or osteoporosis) as well as a decreased absorption of minerals, such as calcium, zinc or magnesium, may occur with a prolonged high-fiber reduction diet. Therefore, do not overindulge.

For those of you who have difficulty counting calories, simply try the following:

1. *Reduce* your usual intake of the following foods by half (50 percent) to three quarters (75 percent). For example, four slices of bread daily becomes a maximum of two, or preferably one slice daily.
   a. All white flour products: bread, pasta, spaghetti, macaroni, roti. Do not eat cakes, cookies or pastries.
   b. Rice.
   c. Fried potatoes. One medium baked potato with skin can be eaten twice weekly.
   d. Avoid fast foods and canned food because of their high calorie and salt content (see Table 3).
2. *Increase* your intake of:
   a. All vegetables, including avocado, which is high in potassium and polyunsaturated fat. Avocado is not fattening as some would have us believe.
   b. All fruits.
   c. Food with high fiber content; except broccoli, turnip greens and alfalfa, which are rich in vitamin K. Small helpings of spinach or cabbage have less vitamin K and can be used.
   d. Fish, chicken, veal, turkey. Fatty fish contain good fats.

In addition, if your blood cholesterol is greater than 240 mg (6 mmol), use only lean cuts of beef or steak twice weekly and only two eggs weekly. If your cholesterol is less than 190 mg (5 mmol), you can have a "nice" steak twice, shrimps once without batter, and three to four eggs weekly.

The combination of foods allowed will afford pleasant-tasting meals that you can tolerate for months to years without depletion of protein, vitamins or minerals. You will lose weight if you combine this diet with one hour of exercise at least five days weekly.

Obesity has been known to be a difficult problem to control. Motivation, willpower and sacrifice are required. You may have greater success if you join a weight loss program or consult with a nutritionist regularly. Though a behavior modification program may help some, to be really successful you need to find a weight loss program that will fit your particular lifestyle and weight loss goals.

You should not use diet plans that recommend low carbohydrates and advise a moderate-to-high fat intake. Some diet recipes reduce carbohydrates, but increase eggs, cheese and meat products. Therefore, an increase in blood cholesterol may occur.

Studies have shown that liquid protein diets have certainly caused deaths and must not be used. Fifty deaths were reported in individuals who were using liquid protein diets. Seventeen of these individuals were known to be healthy, but developed abnormal heart rhythms while on the liquid protein diet. No deaths occurred in a well-supervised study, however, in which about 4,000 individuals were given an adequate amount (70 g) of first-class protein daily, along with a very-low-calorie diet.

OXYGEN

Oxygen is not often required by patients with heart disease except when admitted to hospital because of severe shortness of breath caused by heart failure. Oxygen may be necessary in these patients for a few days only. In patients with chest pain and heart attack, oxygen is given for a few hours only. Heart attacks do not usually cause a lack of oxygen in the blood. In a few patients, heart failure develops but usually clears in a few days. On discharge from hospital, patients with heart disease are not prescribed oxygen at home. Home oxygen is not usually required in heart patients, including those with severe disease. In patients with both heart and lung problems, when shortness of breath is excessive and chronic, home oxygen therapy may be required, if a special blood test of oxygen content of the arterial blood is below 60 mm Hg.

PACEMAKERS

A cardiac pacemaker is an electronic device that delivers electrical stimuli to the heart. It may be necessary to insert a temporary pacemaker in a few patients in whom the heart attack has disturbed the electrical conducting system of the heart.

In about two in every 100 patients with a heart attack, the sinus node pacemaker in the right atrium and the electrical pathway connecting the atrium and the ventricle become damaged and the heart rate becomes very slow (see Fig. 16). The heart rate may fall to less than 36 beats per minute. If the condition does not respond to drugs such as atropine, a temporary pacemaker, which is required only for two to five days, is inserted through a vein (see Fig. 15).

The procedure is a simple one. The temporary pacemaker consists of a pacing wire that is inserted through a vein in the

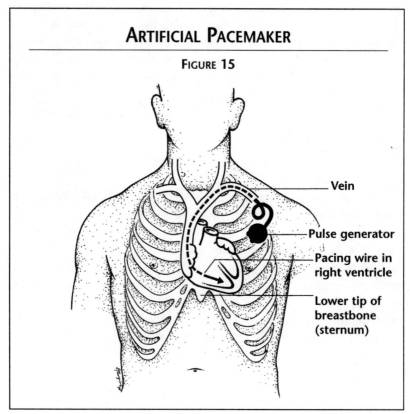

ARTIFICIAL PACEMAKER

FIGURE 15

Vein

Pulse generator

Pacing wire in
right ventricle

Lower tip of
breastbone
(sternum)

neck, usually the subclavian vein. The skin over the vein is infiltrated with a local anesthetic so that the procedure is not painful.
A pacing catheter is threaded through the vein to reach the inside
of the right ventricle. The passage of the pacing catheter is usually
done under fluoroscopic (X-ray) control since the wire is radio-
opaque and can be seen on the X-ray. Occasionally the procedure
is done with the assistance of the electrocardiogram and the final
position of the catheter verified by X-ray. The external end of the
wire catheter is connected to a battery-operated pulse generator
(see Fig. 15). The pulse generator is set, for example, at about 65
beats per minute, and commences pacing if the heartbeat falls
below this set rate. The pacemaker works (fires) only when it is
required, that is, on demand. Complications are very few for the
insertion and maintenance of the pacemaker in the heart for two
to seven days.

PERMANENT PACEMAKER

A pacemaker is often required in the management of patients who
have complete heart block or a condition called sick sinus
syndrome, which we will discuss shortly.

In about one in every 500 patients with a heart attack, the
electrical conducting system is permanently damaged. The heart
rate becomes very slow, less than 36 per minute, and loss of
consciousness may occur. The condition is called heart block
because there is a block of the conduction of electrical impulses
from the atrium through the main electrical tunnel (atrioventricular
node) that transmits the impulses to the ventricle (see Fig. 16).
The atrium normally contracts at 72 beats per minute and in heart
block continues to beat at 72 per minute but the ventricles fail to
receive the message to do the same. Pacemaker cells in the ventricle may create an electrical impulse but beat at a rate less than 36
per minute. Occasionally, in this condition, the ventricles fail to
contract, as there is no electrical stimulus, or the ventricle quivers
(ventricular fibrillation) and loss of consciousness occurs. In such
patients a pacemaker site in the ventricle may suddenly restart the
heart and the patient recovers in a few seconds. A similar condition occurs in individuals who have a rare degenerative disease of
the conduction system; simply, the electrical wires of the heart are
bad, but the heart muscle, coronary arteries and valves are relatively normal. Cases of heart block may also occur in childhood

because of a congenital defect in the conduction system, but fortunately the condition is rare. In patients with degenerative disease of the conduction system and with congenital heart block, the remainder of the heart is completely normal and the insertion of a permanent pacemaker allows for normal activity and life span.

As mentioned above, a permanent pacemaker may also be necessary in patients who have a condition called sick sinus syndrome. In this condition, because of coronary heart disease, the normal sinus node pacemaker may have been destroyed because of lack of blood supply. The heartbeat then becomes erratic; at times, the heart may beat very slowly (36 to 48 per minute) and at other times beats quickly (100 to 150 per minute). The patient may complain of dizziness or transient loss of consciousness (syncope). A permanent pacemaker is inserted and the patient gets complete relief of symptoms if the symptoms were due to a sick sinus node. The condition is rare and is most often seen in individuals over age 65. It is important to document that these symptoms are due to a sick sinus because they can also be caused by several other conditions, including lack of circulation to the brain, that a pacemaker will not help.

WHAT A PACEMAKER WILL NOT DO

1. A pacemaker does not cause the heart muscle to contract more forcefully; therefore, it does not help heart failure except in some cases where a very slow heart rate was contributing to the heart failure.
2. It does not increase the blood supply through the coronary arteries; therefore, it does not help chest pain or angina or prevent a heart attack.
3. A pacemaker does not replace the usual cardiac medications prescribed for various heart conditions. You need to take the medications prescribed by your doctor for heart failure, angina or other conditions that may exist.

A pacemaker is a great device but it does only what it is designed to do. It stimulates the electrical system of the heart so that the heart beats at the correct time and at an appropriate rate. A pacemaker can prolong life provided the problem is that of too slow a heart rate or no heartbeat because of heart block.

TYPES OF PACEMAKERS

There are numerous pacemaker systems on the market. Your cardiologist or cardiac surgeon will choose the one appropriate for you. Usually, the individual requiring a pacemaker is admitted to the hospital. The pacemaker is inserted by a cardiac surgeon and occa sionally by a cardiologist during a simple operation. A pacemaker consists of a heart generator that weighs about 40 grams and is implanted under the skin of the lower abdomen or near the collarbone. The tips (leads) of the pacing wire that emerge from the pacemaker generator are inserted into the vein and threaded through to reach a position inside the right ventricle (see Fig. 15). Another method that is occasionally used attaches the tips of the pacing wire to the outside surface of the right ventricle. A pacemaker with a single wire inserted into the right ventricle is called a ventricular pacemaker. A new brand of pacemaker with certain advantages for some patients utilizes two pacing wires. One is positioned in the right ventricle and the other in the right atrium and is called an atrioventricular pacemaker.

Prior to 1972, a power source for the pacemaker was derived from batteries that were chiefly mercury-zinc. These were heavy and lasted two to four years. Most modern pacemakers are programmable. That is, by placing a device on the skin over the generator, radio signals are delivered to the pacer circuitry. This simple procedure is done in a clinic. The patients are usually followed for six to 12 weeks after the pacemaker is inserted, then twice annually. If signs of power-source depletion are observed, the patient is then seen monthly. Power-source depletion is easily detected as a decrease in rate when the system is monitored by passing a magnet over the generator. Batteries are changed every seven to 10 years depending on the make of the pacemaker. The procedure requires minor surgery. The flap of skin is lifted and the pacemaker generator is replaced. Pacemakers are programmed so that they work only when the patient's heart beats slowly, below the set rate. Current pacemakers are electrically shielded so that it is no longer necessary to avoid electrical equipment as was the case with older pacemaker systems.

ACTIVITIES

Patients are allowed to exercise freely to the extent of major advances in electronics, and now virtually all pacemakers are powered by varieties of lithium batteries. The life of the lithium pacemakers varies from seven to 10 years. Each patient is given a card that documents the type, model, serial number, date of installation and approximate life of the pacemaker.

The patients are strongly advised to attend a pacemaker clinic for follow-up in order to detect the rare occurrence of their tolerance. Many are able to jog one to five miles daily and do similar exercises if angina or heart failure are not present. A patient with a pacemaker can lead a normal life (see Case History of Heart Patient under Heart Attacks).

PALPITATIONS AND ABNORMAL HEART RHYTHMS

The sinus node, a very small group of specialized cells, is located in the upper right corner of the heart (see Fig. 16). The node is about 30 millimeters long by three millimeters thick. Through its genetic code and the influx and efflux of sodium and potassium into its cells, this natural pacemaker spontaneously fires electrical discharges that are conducted through electric cable-like bundles to the atria and ventricles and causes the heart muscle to contract about 70 times a minute. The rate slows or gets faster depending on the needs of the body. The sinus node is like a powerful generator and has complete control of the heart rate. Cells outside the sinus node pacemaker, for example, ventricular muscle cells, possess pacemaker activity that is so weak that the normal electrical discharge from the sinus node suppresses them.

Occasionally, these pacemaker cells may interrupt the normal heartbeat, causing a premature beat, also called an extra beat (see Fig. 16).

The electrical conducting system of the heart is vital to life. Damage to the electrical system can occur when the coronary arteries are blocked and fail to supply sufficient blood to the electrical system as may happen after several heart attacks. The electrical system can also be affected by certain degenerative diseases that cause calcification and hardening (sclerosis) of the bundles, and this may interrupt the electrical discharge.

PALPITATIONS, PREMATURE BEATS, IRREGULAR BEATS

The word "palpitation" is used by doctors and by some patients to describe the heartbeat when it is fast, pounding, skipping, or irregular. *A patient posed the following question:* I am 28 and have a problem with a heartbeat pause. This problem comes and goes and may result in five to 10 pauses each minute. Sometimes my heart feels as if it makes an extra beat. If I lie down, the irregularity seems more pronounced. I went to my family doctor, who found nothing wrong. My doctor concluded that these pauses were caused by too much adrenaline in the blood. Could you tell me more about this, the possible causes, cures and long-term harm to the heart? We answered this question as follows: A heartbeat pause is due to an extra beat (extrasystole), medically termed a premature beat (see Fig. 16). Premature beats may originate in the top chamber of the heart. These are referred to as atrial premature beats and they are of no significance if they occur in a normal heart. If they occur in the lower chamber, or ventricle, they are called ventricular premature beats. Patients perceive the abnormal heart rhythm as either an extra beat or a pause. An individual may state, "My heart skipped a beat." The extra heartbeat nearly always becomes more prominent when the heart slows while sitting or lying. When the heart speeds up during walking or other activities, the extra beats are often suppressed by the normal beats. Movement of the body also prevents the sensation of the stronger heartbeat.

Premature beats may be due to either heart disease or extracardiac conditions, but often, they have no definable cause. Heart diseases that affect the heartbeat include disturbance of the blood supply to the heart due to coronary heart disease; diseases of the heart valves, usually due to prior rheumatic fever and a common condition called mitral valve prolapse. Valve problems are easily excluded by a physician, who can hear murmurs or clicks when listening with the stethoscope. Echocardiography (cardiac ultrasound) can clarify the cause. Heart muscle diseases (cardiomyopathy) are fortunately rare. Alcohol abuse can, now and then, cause a cardiomyopathy. Viruses that cause a flu-like illness can produce microscopic scars in the heart muscle (myocarditis) that may trigger extra beats. Myocarditis can be difficult to exclude if

ELECTRICAL SYSTEM OF THE HEART

FIGURE 16

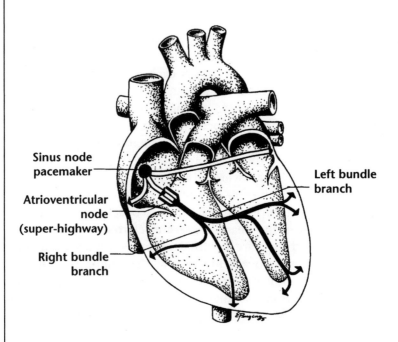

Sinus node pacemaker

Left bundle branch

Atrioventricular node (super-highway)

Right bundle branch

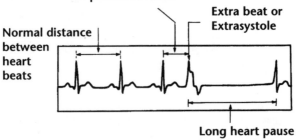

Beat comes too early = premature beat

Extra beat or Extrasystole

Normal distance between heart beats

Long heart pause or skipped beat

The Electrocardiogram picks up the heart's electrical impulses transmitted through the skin of the chest. Premature beat is synonymous with terms extra beat, extrasystole, heart pause or skipped beats.

the patient is not seen during the acute phase.

Investigations of extra beats should include blood tests (to exclude anemia, a low serum potassium or thyroid overactivity), chest X-ray, echocardiography, Holter monitor (24-hour ECG recording) and a stress test.

Extracardiac conditions include alcohol, smoking, stimulants such as caffeine, amphetamines (diet pills) and nicotinic acid in megavitamins and several drugs. In susceptible individuals, disturbances of the heartbeat (arrhythmias) are more common 12 to 24 hours after alcohol consumption. Other causes include low oxygen in the blood due to lung diseases and thyroid overactivity.

Premature or extra beats commonly occur in young individuals with normal hearts and cause no harmful effects. In the normal heart, they bear no relation to heart attacks, sudden cardiac death or heart failure, and they do not produce harm to the heart.

Drug treatment is not indicated for patients with a normal heart since the side effects outweigh the benefits. Some patients, who are terribly bothered by numerous extra beats in the presence of a normal heart or mitral valve prolapse, respond to beta-blockers. Five to 15 pauses or premature beats per minute in a normal heart is of no significance and requires no drug treatment.

Patients may have an extra beat that occurs after each normal heartbeat and more commonly after two normal beats. Those who have episodes of very fast heartbeat, usually 150 to 180 beats per minute, may have a condition known as paroxysmal atrial tachycardia. If episodes are frequent, drug treatment may be necessary.

There is no conclusive evidence that excessive adrenaline triggers paroxysmal atrial tachycardia. In a few individuals, excessive adrenaline may play a role during stress or during a heart attack. Beta-blockers can be useful when stress or heart attack precipitates extra beats. Excessive adrenaline is liberated in the heart muscle during a heart attack and does increase the occurrence of premature beats and other abnormal heart rhythms.

In the majority of individuals with premature beats, there is no good reason why they should occur at a particular time of the day or month. We explain to our patients that it is like having an itchy spot in the elbow crease that can come and go a few times per month or year. A microscopic area in the heart has an "itchy spot." We have never heard of an itch that killed anyone! Several studies have utilized the 24-hour Holter monitor to show that more than 66 percent of normal individuals studied have extra beats arising from the ventricles (ventricular premature beats). We emphasize that unless serious heart disease is present, all the bumpings, flutterings, thumpings and irregular beats can be ignored.

TACHYCARDIA

This is the term used by the medical profession to describe a fast heart rate, greater than 100 per minute. We will describe five types of tachycardia:

1. Sinus tachycardia
2. Atrioventricular nodal reentrant tachycardia, formerly paroxysmal atrial tachycardia (PAT)
3. Atrial fibrillation
4. Wolff-Parkinson-White Syndrome (WPW)
5. Ventricular tachycardia

Sinus Tachycardia

When the fast beat arises from the normal sinus node pacemaker, it is called a sinus tachycardia, which is a normal occurrence during exercise, infections causing fever, anxiety states and thyroid overactivity.

Atrioventricular Nodal Reentrant Tachycardia (AVNRT), Formerly Known as Paroxysmal Atrial Tachycardia (PAT)

This is one of the commonest abnormal tachycardias occurring in young healthy adults. Pacemaker cells outside the sinus node or a circuit in the atrioventricular (AV) node commences an electrical discharge and takes over the heart rhythm for a few minutes to a few hours. The commonest type of paroxysmal tachycardia is one originating in the AV node (see Fig. 15) and is called atrioventricular nodal reentrant tachycardia (AVNRT). We have used the term PAT to embrace AVNRT, but these two have subtle differences. Most cases called PAT are truly AVNRT. The term PAT was introduced more than 50 years ago.

One of our patients, Mrs. M.H., age 76, can recall having PAT from age 22. Without warning, she would feel a sudden pounding of the heart. The beats were so rapid that it was difficult to count them. She would try certain maneuvers such as lying down, walking around or taking a warm drink, all to no avail. Attacks would come on once or twice a year; in one year she had five episodes; the duration of the attacks was usually from several minutes to three or four hours.

She was age 38 when she presented herself at the emergency room because the particular episode had gone on for more than three hours. The episode stopped a few minutes after she came to the emergency room. She was informed that she had PAT, but she truly had AVNRT. Her attacks have a typical sudden onset with a rapid heart rate and abrupt cessation. Occasionally she feels dizzy, as if she is about to faint, but she has never really lost consciousness. We reassured her that PAT nearly always occurs in a normal heart and this was the situation in her case. In addition, in a normal heart, PAT does not cause heart failure or angina, nor does it lead to a heart attack. She was at that time being treated with quinidine and had nausea and diarrhea. We discontinued the quinidine and advised her how she might suppress the attacks through the use of certain maneuvers that increase the activity of the vagus nerve. The vagus nerve is like the reins of a horse; it slows the heart and keeps it in check.

Simple maneuvers to suppress PAT (we are truly describing AVNRT in this patient) are:

1. Gagging: putting a finger at the back of the tongue to produce retching.
2. Holding both nostrils tightly and breathing out against the resistance for about 30 seconds.
3. Holding the breath and immersing the face in cold water for about 10 seconds.

She was warned not to apply pressure on the eyeball. This was used by some several years ago, but it is not recommended since detachment of the retina may occur.

On a few occasions we were able to stop her attacks in the emergency room by massaging her right carotid artery in the neck (carotid sinus) for three to six seconds. This stimulates the vagus nerve and suddenly stops the abnormal fast heart rhythm in more than 50 percent of individuals. The technique should not be tried until the patient is hooked up to a cardiac monitor or electrocardiogram. If these facilities are not available, someone needs to listen to the heartbeat while the doctor presses the carotid sinus.

The technique is not used in individuals over age 60 or in those whose carotid arteries are known to have obstruction by atheroma.

Mrs. M. H.'s attacks became more frequent after age 50. She was tried on digoxin, which was a 75 percent success for one to two years. She later required a beta-blocker, which often helps this situation. You will recall that beta-blockers slow the heart rate. Very rarely a combination of digoxin and beta-blocker is necessary to suppress attacks, and this was tried with success for one to two years. Finally, at age 51 she was tried on the beta-blocker acebutolol alone and this was effective. At age 76, except for two or three one-hour episodes per year, her heart remains normal.

The majority of patients with AVNRT get immediate relief in the emergency room when given a calcium antagonist, verapamil, intravenously. The drug cannot be used, however, in individuals who have heart failure or who have a weak heart muscle, because it can precipitate heart failure in such cases. *A new drug, adenosine, is safer and as effective as verapamil.* Adenosine given intravenously corrects the condition within a few seconds, but the drug is much more expensive than verapamil.

Atrial Fibrillation

Atrial fibrillation is the most common persistent abnormal heart rhythm requiring treatment by doctors. The heart beats are completely irregular. The condition usually occurs after age 30 and can be due to previous rheumatic fever that damaged the valve and left scars in the atria. The atrium beats extremely fast, about 400 to 500 times per minute; however, the impulses that arise from these beats, occurring outside the sinus node, cannot all pass through the atrioventricular node. The atrioventricular (AV) node is like a superhighway that leads to the ventricle (see Fig. 16). At most, it can manage to carry 200 to 220 cars. Therefore, 400 or more cars cause a traffic jam, and in an erratic fashion, only a few can reach the ventricle. The ventricles therefore beat at 120 to 200 per minute, but very irregularly. The condition is usually treated with digoxin, which causes a block in the superhighway tollgate (atrioventricular node) and allows less traffic to reach the ventricles. Instead of the ventricles beating at 120 to 200 per minute, therefore, they beat at 60 to 100 per minute. A beta-blocker is often given once daily with digoxin or alone to slow the very fast heart rate.

Atrial fibrillation can on rare occasions occur during a heart attack and in other conditions such as an overactive thyroid (thyrotoxicosis) and occasionally in severe lung diseases when there is chronic oxygen lack. The condition is usually kept under control and patient's activities are not curtailed. If there is no serious underlying heart disease, life span can be normal. The condition is not to be confused with the dangerous ventricular fibrillation. In patients with heart disease, atrial fibrillation may precipitate heart failure. Also, in patients with murmurs caused by valve disease, atrial fibrillation is a common cause of strokes. Therefore, anticoagulants (blood thinners) are given to prevent strokes.

Wolff-Parkinson-White Syndrome (WPW)

This is a form of tachycardia that is similar to AVNRT but is less common. Individuals age 15 to 40 may get severe tachycardia. In this condition, there is an extra electrical bundle running from the atrium to the ventricle. Conduction of impulses occurs much more quickly through this accessory or *anomalous* bundle, whereas the atrioventricular node tends to impede traffic and so maintain a slow heart rate. The heart is otherwise normal. This condition has a typical ECG appearance and during attacks the heart rate may be as fast as 200 to 250 per minute. Special drugs are now available to treat this abnormal rhythm, and in some cases, the accessory bundle may have to be divided by a special nonsurgical ablation technique that uses radio-frequency. Recent advances have made this procedure highly successful.

Ventricular Tachycardia

By definition, more than three premature ventricular beats occurring together constitutes ventricular tachycardia. This is a serious abnormal heart rhythm and occurs mainly in patients with severe coronary artery disease or severe disease of the heart muscle. The heartbeat is regular but fast, between 120 and 200 per minute, and usually the diagnosis is easily known from the ECG appearance. During a heart attack, ventricular tachycardia may occur and it is usually treated with a drug called lidocaine, followed by other drugs to suppress this rhythm. If success is not obtained, the patient's abnormal heart rhythm is converted to normal sinus rhythm with the use of a cardioverter, which delivers small electrical shocks to the heart. Such a cardioversion is carried out in the emergency room or the coronary care unit after the patient has had sedation with Valium or another similar sedative. The patient therefore feels no pain. Frequent bothersome ventricular premature beats and nonsustained ventricular tachycardia are treated best with beta-blockers, and in some, amiodarone may be necessary.

Drug Treatment

Digoxin (Lanoxin)

Digoxin is used to treat patients with recurrent attacks of atrioventricular nodal reentrant tachycardia (AVNRT). The drug is used daily for a prolonged period, and recurrent attacks are prevented in more than 75 percent of individuals. The important role of digoxin in slowing the heart rate in patients with atrial fibrillation with or without heart failure has been discussed.

Beta-Blockers

Beta-blockers are occasionally used to treat AVNRT and are successful in more than 60 percent of cases. As well, the drugs can be used to treat bothersome ventricular premature beats when they are associated with increased secretion of adrenaline and in individuals who have a minor defect of the mitral valve, termed mitral valve prolapse. The drugs have a beneficial effect on ventricular premature beats produced during or following a heart attack. They are the only safe drugs that have been proven to prevent sudden cardiac deaths and heart attacks.

Several other drugs are used to treat more difficult and serious heart rhythm disorders. Most of these drugs have serious side effects, are only 60 to 80 percent effective in controlling the disturbance, and they do not prevent death. Thus, doctors are not keen to treat premature beats unless they are associated with serious heart disease. In such patients, when premature beats are numerous with runs of four or more occurring together for more than 30 seconds, drugs are usually tried.

Sotalol (Sotacor)

Sotalol is the most effective beta-blocker available for the treatment of abnormal heart rhythms. The action is prolonged and the drug is effective when taken once daily. It is not affected by smoking.

Dosage: 80 mg once or twice daily for four weeks, then 160 mg once daily, maximum 240 mg daily.

Amiodarone (Cordarone)

The drug is effective in suppressing life-threatening abnormal heart rhythms and is approved only for treating recurrent episodes of sustained ventricular tachycardia.

Advice and Adverse Effects

The drug's major toxicity includes deposits of granules in the cornea, fibrosis of the lung in about 5 percent and grayish blue discoloration of the skin with prolonged use at high doses.

Amiodarone must not be used in combination with verapamil. Interaction may occur when used concomitantly with quinidine, digoxin and oral anticoagulants such as warfarin.

Disopyramide

This drug has similar effects as quinidine. It is useful in the emergency treatment of ventricular tachycardia when given intravenously. Oral treatment suppresses premature beats in about 50 percent of cases.

Advice and Adverse Effects

The drug should not be used in patients with heart failure or poor heart muscle function since it can precipitate heart failure. The drug is contraindicated in individuals with glaucoma, kidney failure, low blood pressure and enlargement of the prostate because urinary retention can be precipitated. The drug must not be used in combination with verapamil.

Lidocaine (Lignocaine)

This drug is used intravenously in emergency situations and is effective in suppressing ventricular tachycardia and serious premature beats. This relatively nontoxic drug is discussed under Heart Attacks.

Mexiletine

This drug is more effective than disopyramide. It suppresses complex abnormal heart rhythms but it has not improved survival rate.

Advice and Adverse Effects

Mexiletine is contraindicated in patients with low blood pressure. The dose must be reduced if kidney failure is present. Side effects include slowing of the pulse, stomach problems, confusional states, double vision and disturbance in walking (ataxia). The drug is therefore reserved for the treatment of life-threatening arrhythmias.

Procainamide

Procainamide has similarities to the well-known quinidine. It is of value when given intravenously in the emergency management of ventricular tachycardia, that is not responsive to lidocaine. When used orally it has a variable effect. It is less effective than quinidine or disopyramide and when used for longer than six months, patients can develop joint pains and fever (lupus erythematosus). As well, although very rare, the white blood cells can be damaged (agranulocytosis).

The drug should not be used in patients with low blood pressure, severe heart failure and myasthenia gravis.

Quinidine

The use of quinidine has greatly decreased since the advent of other antiarrhythmic agents. The drug suppresses premature beats in about 60 percent of cases but is only partially effective with life-threatening arrhythmias. Because of rare but serious side effects, the use of the drug is questionable.

Advice and Adverse Effects

Quinidine can precipitate ventricular fibrillation, which is the most dangerous abnormal heart rhythm. It does not seem reasonable to give priority to a drug that may increase the risk of ventricular fibrillation and death. Quinidine may precipitate ventricular tachycardia and cardiac arrest.

Quinidine increases the level of digoxin in the blood and when used concomitantly, care is necessary with digoxin and anticoagulants such as warfarin.

Conclusion

We have a long way to go in the management of simple premature beats, more complex extra beats, ventricular tachycardia and the prevention of ventricular fibrillation, which is the cause of death in many heart patients.

Questions still to be answered include the following:

1. Are the drugs effective in suppressing the abnormal rhythm?
2. Do they prevent ventricular fibrillation and prolong life, especially during and after a heart attack? Only beta-blockers have been proven. Amiodarone appears to be partially effective but causes serious side effects.
3. How serious are their side effects, including the precipitation of more dangerous heart rhythms? Many patients have died due to the use of drugs such as encainide, flecainide and moricizine.
4. Is their use justified in the given individual?

At present, partial success with the use of complex drug combinations in the seriously ill has been achieved, yet life has not been prolonged. In addition to toxicity, several visits to the doctor and cost must be justified.

Automatic Implantable Cardioverter Defibrillator

When life is severely threatened by the recurrence of abnormal heart rhythms that have caused cardiac arrest or recurrent sustained ventricular tachycardia, the automatic implantable cardioverter defibrillator has a role in selected patients. Recent advances in this area allow a ray of hope. Dr. Saksena in New Jersey has introduced a nonsurgical technique for implanting the automatic cardioverter defibrillator. Clinical trials have shown this to be a highly successful breakthrough.

SMOKING AND HEART DISEASE

If cigarette smoking were eliminated, about a quarter of a million lives now lost because of cardiovascular disease could be saved yearly in North America. Each year, lung cancer causes about 80,000 deaths. Smoking causes most cases of lung cancer, which is becoming the leading cause of death from cancer in women.

Nonsmoking men age 45 to 55 are 10 times less likely to have a fatal or nonfatal heart attack than heavy smokers. The Multiple Risk Factor Intervention Trial showed that men at high risk who stopped smoking had a significant reduction in their mortality.

The detrimental effects of cigarette smoking were widely advertised in the mid-1970s, and since then more than 20 million North Americans have stopped smoking. Smoking has increased in teenagers and women, however, resulting in little change in the overall number of smokers. Heart attacks are rare in women age 40 to 48 but in women of this age who use oral contraceptives and smoke, the heart attack rate is increased.

Low-nicotine, low-tar brands or filter cigarettes do not decrease the risk of coronary heart disease, although the risk of lung cancer may be decreased. Filter cigarettes deliver more carbon monoxide and cause a higher incidence of coronary heart disease than do plain cigarettes.

If you cannot quit but can change to a pipe, this will certainly decrease the risk, since studies have shown that pipe and cigar smokers have only a slight increase in cardiac death. You must not smoke Cheroot, since a higher risk of heart attacks was found to occur in Danish Cheroot smokers than in cigarette smokers.

EFFECTS OF COMPONENTS OF CIGARETTE SMOKE

Tobacco smoke contains more than 4,000 components. Some of these are nicotine, carbon monoxide, ammonia, benzene, nitrobenzene, phenol, 2,4 dimethylphenol, acetaldehyde, hydrogen cyanide, toluene and O-cresol. Most studies have been done on nicotine and various gases, in particular, carbon monoxide (CO). Although the effects of the many constituents of smoke are not understood, the effects of nicotine and CO are well documented.

Nicotine

Nicotine stimulates the adrenal glands to put out excessive adrenaline and noradrenaline. The higher the nicotine concentration inhaled, the greater the outpouring of adrenaline. If someone puts a gun to your head, you need all the adrenaline and noradrenaline that your adrenals and nerves can produce to enable you to fight or run. So adrenaline is great stuff, but it has many harmful effects. The heart rate and blood pressure increase, which means more work for the heart. The heart muscle will also require a bigger supply of oxygen. The platelets become sticky and may clump onto the surface of atheromatous plaques in one of your coronary arteries and a heart attack can occur.

Nicotine, by increasing the heart rate and blood pressure, can increase the frequency and duration of chest pain in those who have angina.

Nicotine can and does increase the excitability of heart muscle, causing premature beats that can lead to serious disturbance in heart rhythm (arrhythmias). Sudden cardiac death is more common in heavy cigarette smokers. In individuals with seizures, the brain cells have a threshold level at which seizures occur. If this threshold is not reached, seizures do not occur. Drugs including alcohol decrease this threshold and seizures are more easily produced, but we can prevent seizures by elevating the threshold. Drugs used to treat epilepsy, for example phenytoin (Dilantin), increase the threshold, therefore preventing seizures. Two products of cigarette smoke, nicotine and carbon monoxide, decrease the ventricular fibrillation threshold of heart muscle. The ventricular fibrillation threshold is decreased if the heart muscle is suddenly deprived of blood, or exposed to high concentrations of adrenaline, noradrenaline and other drugs. During a heart attack, high amounts of noradrenaline are found in and around the damaged muscle and can cause ventricular fibrillation. During ventricular fibrillation the muscle no longer contracts, but quivers. Therefore, the heart is really at a standstill and no blood is being pumped. The heart stops beating, the brain dies; thus there is heart and brain death.

The ventricular fibrillation threshold is slightly increased by only one or two available heart drugs. Beta-blockers counteract the effects of adrenaline and noradrenaline at the cell surface and increase the ventricular fibrillation threshold. We would like to emphasize that since 50 years of research on heart disease have yielded so few useful drugs, we have to salvage every possible assistance from nondrug treatment. We hope that this explanation will help you to motivate yourself to stop smoking.

Smokers are inhaling two dangerous compounds, carbon monoxide and nicotine, as well as other gases that decrease the ventricular fibrillation threshold and therefore are capable of causing death. *Quitting is the one way that you can prevent your death.* But we agree, you must be convinced that it is dangerous to smoke so as to be sufficiently motivated to quit. Beware! Lung cancer is common, but heart attacks are very common. There are some of us, the lucky ones, who are immune to all types of knocks including an outpouring of adrenaline, be it from stress, cigarettes or other stimuli generated by the body. Therefore, do not use the excuse that your uncle or your aunt or your friends smoke two packs of cigarettes daily and are still living at an age greater than 80. Unfortunately we do not have methods to pick out the 40 or 50 percent of the population that will respond badly to smoking, stress or a high consumption of saturated fats. Note that hypertension was not listed, as it is a specific disease; we can determine those who have it, and its effects can be documented as well as prevented. Stress, cigarette smoking and high saturated fat intake are not diseases, and only some individuals exposed to all three factors will develop ill effects. Therefore, it is difficult to talk about prevention unless you understand exactly what is at stake.

It is easy to write and talk about prevention programs, yet it is difficult for many individuals and families to diet and reduce blood cholesterol. Stress is usually inevitable and only a few learn how to live with stress. Discontinuation of smoking, however, only takes the effort of one person. You are the one! Smoking is a preventable risk factor. Recognize this, *stop cold turkey* and save yourself. No one can do it for you.

Carbon Monoxide

The hemoglobin of red blood cells transports oxygen to all cells and tissues of the body. Hemoglobin clings to carbon monoxide about 200 times more readily than the oxygen circulating in the blood. In this situation oxygen clings strongly to whatever hemoglobin it can find, and less oxygen is released to the cells. Carbon monoxide combines with hemoglobin to form a compound called carboxyhemoglobin. The tissues, therefore, including the heart muscle cells, are deprived of oxygen. This is particularly important if the cells are already undernourished and lack oxygen because of severe narrowing of the coronary arteries by atheromatous plaques. These plaques are present in more than 50 percent of North Americans age 35 and over. Only about 30 percent of the adult population are spared from the dreadful atheromatous blockage in arteries that cause coronary heart disease (see Fig. 1).

Carboxyhemoglobin likely causes the wall of the arteries to be more permeable to fats including cholesterol, and this can speed up atheroma formation. Individuals with carboxyhemoglobin levels greater than 5 percent are 21 times more likely to develop heart attacks or poor circulation in the arteries of the legs than individuals with levels less than 3 percent. There is scientific evidence indicating that heavy cigarette smokers are subjected to eight times the carbon monoxide exposure allowed in industry. *You will certainly not stay in a car parked in a closed garage with the engine running knowing the danger of carbon monoxide is death. Do you prefer slow death?*

High-nicotine or nonnicotine cigarettes produce the same amount of carbon monoxide. Stickiness of the platelets is also increased by carbon monoxide, thus increasing the chance of clotting in the coronary arteries. The ventricular fibrillation threshold of heart muscle and its electrical tissues is reduced by carbon monoxide; thus sudden death may not be a mystery. Carbon monoxide is more important than nicotine in causing complications of coronary heart disease, but the two components and many others likely work in concert to orchestrate your departure from this earth.

SMOKING AND CHEST PAIN

In conditions such as angina, where oxygen supply to the heart muscle is low, the frequency and severity of chest pain may be increased by cigarettes. Nicotine causes a slight increase in blood pressure and heart rate. Therefore, the heart muscle demands more oxygen. Thus, the combination of carbon monoxide and nicotine increases the bad effects. Patients with angina who are smokers develop chest pain at lower levels of exercise.

Other components of cigarette smoking include a glycoprotein that is highly allergenic and may cause shortness of breath, asthmatic attacks or eye irritation. In addition, the glycoprotein is believed to cause damage to the lining of arteries and an increase in atherosclerosis.

HABITUATION

This is a major problem because nicotine is a potent chemical that has been conclusively shown to produce addiction and dependence. The smoker will go to extremes to purchase his or her cigarettes and ensure that they are readily available. The craving and hunger can be satisfied by smoking a cigarette or by chewing nicotine-containing gum, wearing a nicotine patch or by an injection of nicotine. Note that some heavy smokers who stop *cold turkey* do not get symptoms of withdrawal, and you may be one of the lucky.

IMPOTENCE

Smoking appears to cause a constriction of small penile arteries and may be implicated as one of the many factors responsible for impotence in some individuals.

EFFECTS ON BYSTANDERS

Inhalation of cigarette smoke by nonsmokers is certainly a concern. The smoke from smoldering cigarettes contains a high concentration of carbon monoxide; smoke exhaled by cigarette smokers in a ventilated or nonventilated room contains enough harmful constituents to cause an increase in heart rate, blood pressure and carboxyhemoglobin content of the blood of your spouse, children, friends or bystanders with angina. Therefore it is vital for the public and the various levels of government to insist on nonsmoking areas in all enclosed spaces.

HOW TO STOP SMOKING

This is a fisherman's story. Everyone who has stopped smoking has his or her own story and will usually try to convince others by telling the awful tale, but with very little effect. We do not pretend to have answers and will not try to give you a plan of how to stop smoking, but will offer a few tips.

Motivation is the key, and this may be achieved by clearly understanding the dangers of cigarette smoking. Nicotine is bad but carbon monoxide is worse. *You must bring yourself to believe that cigarette smoking produces enough carbon monoxide to shorten your life span.* You know that carbon monoxide from motor vehicle exhaust is dangerous and can cause death. It is only a matter of how quickly death will occur. You may knock 20 years off your life if you smoke more than 20 cigarettes daily. Quitting is difficult since nicotine is an addictive chemical. It is best to stop *cold turkey* or reduce to 10 cigarettes daily for a few weeks, then switch to a low-nicotine brand for two weeks, then stop. A nicotine patch can be helpful at this stage.

It is particularly hard to get teenagers to stop smoking. The emphasis should be to carefully motivate 10- to 16-year-olds in schools so that they do not start smoking, or give up the habit of smoking two to 10 cigarettes daily since this will soon build up to a larger amount per day. Carefully planned audiovisual programs for class sessions are necessary. These programs must give scientific details including the hazards of the carbon monoxide content of cigarette smoke. We feel that the message regarding carbon monoxide and decrease in ventricular fibrillation threshold is a fruitful area on which to base solid reasoning with the seven- to 17-year-old. Audiovisual programs and antismoking literature should incorporate this message. In addition, the videotapes should incorporate the short-term and long-term benefits of not smoking, the incidence of chronic bronchitis, emphysema, lung cancer and heart attacks. Posters that show a nonsmoking sign with words such as "We urge you not to smoke; beware of the dangers of cigarettes" are not enough to motivate teenagers or seasoned smokers. Nicotine is an addicting drug, and mere words and posters cannot assist the addict. To state that nicotine is addicting seems to carry little weight.

Schools that do not have efficiently run nonsmoking programs are certainly not playing their role in the community. School principals should encourage a student body to organize a nonsmoking campaign and should provide the videotape programs. Advice to children is best given by fellow teenagers who are highly motivated and not by teachers or parents. Peer pressure is always effective. The incidence of smoking was reduced in seventh-grade students by using peer role models and active individual role playing. Teenagers are very keen on a ban on nuclear weapons. They are afraid of a nuclear war that would kill millions. The audiovisual programs and circulated leaflets must show that cigarette smoking kills more than a quarter of a million North Americans yearly, therefore five million deaths in 20 years. This is a real-life situation that is as dangerous as a nuclear war that may never occur. Teenagers cannot prevent a nuclear war, but the good news is that teenagers can prevent the deaths of millions by never getting into the habit of smoking.

Parents are very eager to influence their children. **The smoking parent by stopping smoking can influence his or her children,** especially if they are made aware of the facts outlined in this chapter.

As a bonus, the nonsmoker feels and breathes better and has less difficulty during exercise. At last there is no more dizziness, lightheartedness, mental blocks or bad breath, which means a better kiss for the teenager. In addition (or as a bonus), the individual drastically reduces the risk of having a fatal or nonfatal heart attack, or chronic bronchitis, emphysema or lung cancer.

Some techniques to assist with stopping smoking include the following:

- Participation in stop-smoking clinics and other group programs that emphasize educational and behavioral modification.
- Nicotine chewing gum, patches or tablets, which are of value and should be tried.
- Hypnosis, which may be of value to some individuals.
- Help Health Programs. The American Cancer Society's "I quit kit" with its seven-day program is useful, as well as the National Cancer Institute's "Helping smokers quit kit." (Ask your doctor to obtain a kit for you.) You must develop substitutes; for example, if you feel an urge to smoke, get up, take a walk, talk to someone or get your favorite book. It is important to engage in an exercise program or at least a half-hour brisk walk twice daily and restrict carbohydrates to prevent weight gain.

Congratulations, you have quit! Your smoker's hacking cough will disappear, and your sense of smell and taste will return, and you have added several years to your life.

STRESS AND HEART DISEASE

Stress is not really nervous tension, so we will not dwell on the subject of nervousness and chronic anxiety, the cause of which must be determined and removed. Damaging or unpleasant stress, as Hans Selye states, is "stress with distress and this is always disagreeable." Although stress can be associated with pleasant situations, it is more often produced in the individual by unpleasant stimuli. The word "stress" is derived from the Old French and Middle English words for "distress"; the first syllable was lost over the years.

There is no doubt that stress is awful. With the exception of severe pain and death, severe stress with distress is one of the most difficult situations we have to face.

Stress produces well-known reactions in the body, in particular, an increase in blood pressure, and causes small blood particles (platelets) to become sticky. The platelet particles stick together to form clumps or sludge, which can lead to formation of a blood clot in the coronary artery.

Trauma to your arteries wreaks havoc like a silent curse, a silent killer. During the stress reaction, the arteries constrict under the influence of adrenaline; consequently both systolic and diastolic blood pressure increase. If your blood pressure is usually 120/80, it can go up to 160/90, or from 145/95 to as high as 190/110. These elevated pressures, lasting only minutes, are injurious to the arteries, and when combined with the effects of excess adrenaline, causing platelet sludging in the arteries, we see the death toll from heart attacks rising.

How does stress cause heart pain (angina) and damage to the heart and arteries? When the coronary arteries are narrowed by plaques of atheroma, chest pain may occur (see Angina and Fig. 1). Chest pain is made worse by exertion such as walking up a hill. Pain at rest may occur, however, if the patient faces sudden emotional upset. The individual may feel a distress in the chest.

Stress causes adrenaline and noradrenaline release. These stress hormones cause the heart rate and blood pressure to increase, giving the heart more work to do (see Fig. 17). In some patients, adrenaline may cause platelets to clump onto plaques of atheroma,

STRESS AND THE HEART

FIGURE 17

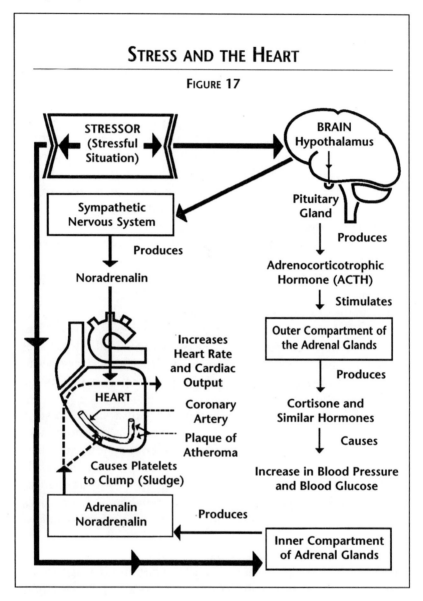

thus causing oxygen lack to that segment of heart muscle. This oxygen lack may or may not produce chest pain.

Moderate stress associated with simple daily activities can decrease the blood supply to the heart muscle in patients with coronary heart disease. In a study of 16 patients who had angina, the moderate stress of mental arithmetic caused oxygen lack to the heart muscle (myocardial ischemia) similar to that produced by exercise (see Fig. 18). In these patients a radioisotope material (rubidium-82) was injected into a vein, and when it reached the heart muscle, photographs were taken. The dark areas in Figure 18 represent the uptake of blood supply to the heart muscle. When the supply of blood is decreased, the area of muscle is poorly supplied with blood, the presence of the radioisotope, rubidium-82, is reduced and the area of darkness is diminished. The simple stress of mental arithmetic causes lack of blood to the heart muscle.

In a similar experiment, a patient who was having catheterization of his heart (coronary arteriogram) was asked to do mental arithmetic, was asked to think of a past stressful situation, and was shown the result of his catheter studies. His heart muscle function was determined during the test and showed no significant change with thinking of past stress, but showed a mild defect during mental arithmetic and severe defects in muscle function during the explanation and viewing of the findings of his heart catheter test. A stressful situation causes the "emotional center" in the brain to trigger certain reactions (Figure 17). The hypothalamus sends signals to the pituitary gland and sympathetic nervous system, which leads to secretion of "stress hormones," cortisone, adrenaline, and noradrenaline. Cortisone causes an increase in blood glucose and an increase in blood pressure.

As a result of a stressful situation (stressor), the inner compartment of the adrenal glands pours out adrenaline and noradrenaline and these compounds are involved in the "fight or flight" reaction.

The external stimulus (stressor) is usually a condition that produces anger, fear, anxiety, deprivation and the like. Common stressors include the death of a spouse, conflicts with others, and projects requiring a deadline. Very often the stressor consists of "words" that are interpreted by the individual as harsh or hurtful, resulting in anger, hostility, humiliation or resentment.

The body reacts in the same way regardless of the type or source of stress or unexpressed anger. An argument with the boss, fellow workers, your spouse or others is the same as if you are being chased by an assailant. The fight for so-called prestige, recognition and survival at work or at home goes on daily, and for many years you may bear the brunt of the attack.

You are riled to the point of bursting and the adrenaline has been poured. Visualize the adrenaline as little death potions that one may drink at work and for some, unfortunately, at home. Adrenaline is helpful in some situations; for example, when you want to flee from a charging bull or an assailant. These

THE HEART UNDER STRESS

FIGURE 18

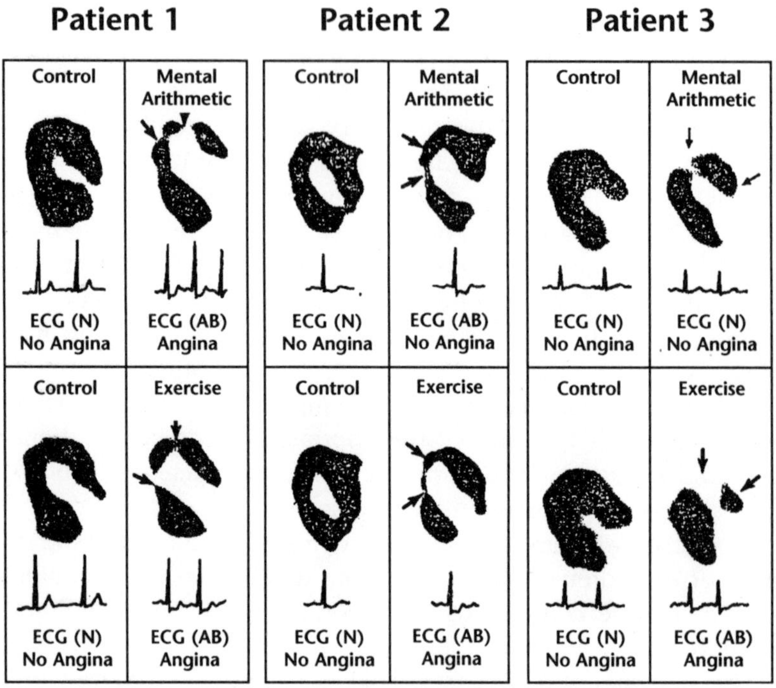

Patient 1	Patient 2	Patient 3

Control	Mental Arithmetic	Control	Mental Arithmetic	Control	Mental Arithmetic
ECG (N) No Angina	ECG (AB) Angina	ECG (N) No Angina	ECG (AB) No Angina	ECG (N) No Angina	ECG (N) No Angina

Control	Exercise	Control	Exercise	Control	Exercise
ECG (N) No Angina	ECG (AB) Angina	ECG (N) No Angina	ECG (AB) Angina	ECG (N) No Angina	ECG (AB) Angina

Changes in the uptake of rubidium-82 and the electrocardiogram in relation to chest pain before and after mental arithmetic or exercise.

Control scans, dark areas, show normal rubidium-82 uptake by the heart muscle in three patients, indicating normal blood flow.

There are defects in uptake (arrows) with mental arithmetic and exercise, and these changes can be accompanied by ECG changes of oxygen lack to the muscle=ischemia=angina.

N = Normal   AB = Abnormal
Modified from Lancet 2: 1003, 1984 (with permission)

compounds increase the heart rate and blood pressure and increase the supply of blood containing glucose and oxygen to exercising muscles so that you are able to run. An excess of adrenaline, and noradrenaline, can be dangerous since these chemicals can overstimulate the heart, disturb its electrical stability and, on rare occasions, lead to ventricular fibrillation, during which the heart does not contract but quivers. This condition is the usual cause of sudden death. Adrenaline causes a decrease in the ventricular fibrillation threshold and can precipitate ventricular fibrillation and cardiac arrest. Adrenaline causes platelets to clump, and if this occurs on a plaque of atheroma, pain can occur or a clot can develop. These compounds can also cause *spasm of the coronary arteries,* which in turn can produce chest pain and sometimes death, especially if the spasm occurs where the plaque partially blocks the artery.

Heart deaths are due to two major problems:

- Formation of a blood clot at the site of partial blockage by atherosclerosis in a coronary artery.
- Electrical disturbances that cause the heart to quiver and not contract (ventricular fibrillation).

Sudden death is common, and the possibility cannot be excluded that severe acute stress may cause death by initiating a brain-adrenaline-heart interaction (see Fig. 17). The clumping of platelets can enlarge the plaque, and over a period of years, the buildup of clot on a plaque can cause complete obstruction of the artery. Animal experiments lend support to this hypothesis. Rats exposed to sudden trauma such as being plunged into ice water develop blockage of the coronary arteries, which results in damage to the segments of the heart muscle (myocardial infarction). When rats were not physically traumatized, but were stressed with nonphysically traumatic electric shocks, they developed clots in the coronary arteries and died. When rats were pretreated with drugs that prevent platelet clumping, such as aspirin or dipyridamole, and then subjected to similar electric shocks, clots were prevented in the majority. If rats are pretreated with a beta-blocker, which blocks the dangerous effects of adrenaline, ventricular fibrillation is prevented and rats survive.

Experimentally, adrenaline or noradrenaline given intravenously can cause severe electrical disturbances and ventricular fibrillation. During a heart attack, there is an increase in noradrenaline in the heart muscle. When blood flow to the heart is reduced by atherosclerosis of the coronary artery, severe stress can more easily precipitate ventricular fibrillation. There are several reports that document these (see later discussion).

When a coronary artery is suddenly blocked in dogs, severe quivering of the heart occurs in some. When the hypothalamus (in

the brain) and sympathetic nervous system are stimulated to produce noradrenaline at the same time that the coronary artery is
blocked, quivering of the heart frequently occurs. Beta-blocking
drugs block the actions of adrenaline and noradrenaline, and if
dogs are pretreated with these drugs and the coronary artery is then
blocked, the dangerous quivering of the heart can be prevented.

In a study involving 117 patients who were resuscitated from
cardiac arrest, 25 reported that they had severe stress such as job
and family conflicts within the 24 hours prior to the cardiac arrest.
Acute or prolonged (chronic) stress may produce severe damage
to the coronary arteries. You must remember that atheroma of the
arteries commonly produces no symptoms; it is a silent killer. After
many years, a clot develops on a ruptured atheromatous plaque.
There is considerable evidence linking increased stickiness of
platelets to the production of atheroma and blockage of arteries.

STRESS AND SPORTS

Do not push yourself to jog or run. Do it if you feel great and
enjoy it, and don't have to clench your jaws or tighten your facial
muscles. If you have to push yourself to do an additional mile,
then you may secrete excess adrenaline and noradrenaline and
this takes its toll on your cardiovascular system throughout the
years. Similarly, be careful not to be overly competitive when
playing racquet sports. No one gets hurt under age 30, but if you
are more than 40, very competitive vigorous sports such as squash
and racquetball can occasionally hurt your cardiovascular system.

THE SYMPTOMS AND SIGNS OF STRESS

- You immediately feel sweaty, especially on the forehead, on
  the skull, under the armpits and on the palms, owing to the
  presence of excess adrenaline.
- Your heart races and may easily pound.
- You feel an ache in the head and neck, especially in your
  temples or eyes.
- You have a feeling of turmoil, or tightness in the chest or
  stomach. You may feel as if there were butterflies in your
  stomach, or there is a feeling of anguish, terror, fright, restlessness, agitation or tremulousness. You may feel shaky,

jittery or weak all over.

- Your speech is slurred and you feel that you cannot even scream or talk for a few seconds.
- You may feel hostile, violent, full of rage and anger, and ready to fight back.
- You have difficulty sleeping.
- You may experience frequency of urination, indigestion or sometimes diarrhea.

HOW TO HANDLE STRESS

Stress is a part of living and cannot be completely avoided. When you understand how traumatic stress can be to your heart and arteries, you may be motivated to develop techniques to deal with stress.

Stress management is a complex subject, beyond the scope of this book. Therefore, we will not attempt to give specific stress management techniques.

Some of the ways that are indicated to cope with stress include mental diversion, techniques to develop a healthy self-concept, time management, progressive deep relaxation techniques, meditation, biofeedback and exercise.

CONCLUSION

We believe that stress is as important as the major "risk factors," but it is difficult to prove this hypothesis scientifically. Stress, high blood cholesterol, hypertension, smoking and blood-clotting factors work in concert in the genetically susceptible individual to produce atherosclerosis and, finally, a fatal or nonfatal heart attack. A stressor causes the sympathetic nervous system and adrenal glands to secrete stress hormones, which increase the work of the heart, and cause platelet clumping that can sometimes cause a blood clot in the coronary artery. We have outlined how excess adrenaline and noradrenaline alter the electrical stability of the heart, predisposing it to a high risk of a curious quivering (ventricular fibrillation) during which it fails to contract, and sudden death may occur.

Human beings are fortunate that the working of the body is such that the reaction caused by one chemical is often counterbalanced by other chemicals that are produced in the body. Nature does not always win, but it can, with a little help from a friend — you! We strongly urge you to develop strategies that may enable you to deal with various stressful situations. Thus you will be able to handle stress and subdue the brain-adrenaline-heart-artery reaction, described above.

STROKE

A stroke is caused by brain damage that results from obstruction of an artery supplying that area of the brain. Obstruction of the artery is caused by blood clot formation in the artery, often at a point where the artery is narrowed by atherosclerosis (see Atherosclerosis). If part of the brain that controls movement of the hand or leg is involved, then loss of strength or complete paralysis of the arm and/or leg occurs. If the speech area of the brain is involved, speech difficulties become apparent and in some patients, a complete loss of speech occurs.

Some patients have warning attacks of stroke: blindness in one eye with mild weakness and tingling or numbness of the arm, hand or leg on the opposite side to the affected eye. The symptoms and signs may persist for only minutes, but can last up to 24 hours with full recovery and without stroke occurring. These warning attacks are called transient ischemic attacks (TIA). If symptoms and signs last more than 24 hours, a stroke is the usual outcome.

Prevention of this type of stroke caused by clot formation in an artery in the brain can be partially achieved by slightly thinning the blood by aspirin. Excellent control of blood pressure helps to prevent strokes. Success in patients has been achieved with the use of 325 to 650 mg aspirin daily, but a dose as low as 80 mg is usually effective. Aspirin prevents blood particles from sticking together to form small friable clots in the artery. These small friable clots may break off and temporarily block small arteries, causing warning attacks or a small stroke. Patients who cannot take aspirin because of bleeding from the stomach or gut benefit from the use of ticlopidine (Ticlid); this agent may, however, cause damage to white blood cells, albeit rarely.

Strokes are commonly due to obstruction of the carotid arteries in the neck as the artery continues deep to the jawbone and enters the brain. Surgery to clean this artery, endarterectomy, is useful in patients with more than 70 percent obstruction of the carotid artery. A simple test called a carotid Doppler examines the velocity of flow of blood through the carotid artery and gives a reasonable estimate of obstruction: less than 33 percent, non-significant, greater than 50 percent, significant, or greater than 75 percent, severe obstruction. The test is done within minutes as an outpatient and does not require an injection. Before surgery is advised, the result of the Doppler is confirmed by a dye test, carotid angiogram.

A second type of stroke caused by rupture of a small artery in the brain results in hemorrhage into the brain substance with consequent damage of a large area of the brain. This type of stroke has a bad prognosis. Moderate to severe hypertension for several years is the most common cause of cerebral hemorrhage.

In addition, a small aneurysm of an artery at the base of the brain may rupture and bleed into the subarachnoid space around the brain. These small aneurysms are called berry aneurysms and may be due to a developmental defect on the wall of the artery, which stretches, balloons and forms a small aneurysmal dilatation of the artery. The blood from the ruptured aneurysm may damage the brain substance, and the pressure of the blood clot pressing against the brain leads to a rapid loss of consciousness. The condition is called subarachnoid hemorrhage (see Aneurysm).

Considerable brain damage may occur, but urgent surgery to remove the clotted blood that is compressing the brain and to clip the aneurysm is often successful in causing a 75 percent or better recovery. Unfortunately, this type of hemorrhage occurs suddenly in young individuals, aged 25 to 50. A sudden, very severe headache becoming unbearable over minutes to an hour, especially associated with drowsiness or mild confusion, may herald the onset of this type of hemorrhage. Urgent investigation by surgery may prevent disaster. In a few patients, because of recurrent episodes of intense headaches, the diagnosis is made by an angiogram done prior to the rupture of the aneurysm. Clipping the aneurysm is a simple operation because the artery lies outside the brain substance, and is highly successful.

Another form of stroke is caused by a small clot that is present in the chamber of the heart. This clot becomes dislodged and is propelled by the blood into the brain. This process is called an embolus. Clots in the heart may form in patients after a heart attack or in others with a common abnormality of heart rhythm called atrial fibrillation (see Atrial Fibrillation). Aspirin is useful in preventing strokes caused by embolism from the heart up to age 65, but if the heart valves are affected, or the heart is enlarged, more powerful thinning of the blood is necessary with the use of anticoagulants (warfarin, Coumadin); this treatment is more effective than the use of aspirin but carries the risk of bleeding.

TESTS FOR HEART DISEASES

THE ELECTROCARDIOGRAM (ECG)

The ECG at rest in patients with angina is often normal but can show signs of chronic oxygen lack (ischemia) or an old scar of a healed heart attack (myocardial infarct). The ECG may show disturbances of the heart rhythm, i.e., premature beats and electrical disturbances as well as heart enlargement. The ECG is a valuable test for patients with heart disease, but a normal ECG does not mean that the individual does not have angina.

The resting ECG may show the following abnormalities:

- Diagnostic of an acute heart attack in patients with chest pain. The ECG is still the most important test used for the diagnosis of a heart attack. Expensive nuclear scans and blood tests cannot replace the inexpensive ECG.
- An old heart attack, which has caused a residual scar in the heart muscle.
- Acute oxygen lack in patients with unstable angina.
- Chronic ischemic changes due to oxygen lack or changes that indicate that the left ventricle is working under strain.
- Electrical disturbances such as blocks in the electrical bundles, called right or left bundle branch block or heart block.
- Ventricular premature beats and a variety of abnormal heart rhythms that cause palpitations (see Palpitations).
- Enlargement of the left or right ventricle and the left atrium.

- A very weak area or bulge of the heart muscle (aneurysm).
- A very slow heart rate, which may indicate disease of the sinus node generator (pacemaker). If a prior ECG is available, a comparison in pattern is most useful. Therefore, it is wise for heart patients who are traveling outside the country or state to carry an ECG during their travels. This may prevent holdup in emergency rooms and hasten discharge from hospital.
- Several others disturbances are appreciated by a resting ECG. Potassium and calcium lack or excess, digoxin toxicity, pericarditis, athlete's heart, muscle problems and others. Despite the advent of sophisticated and very expensive cardiologic tests, the inexpensive ECG retains its usefulness as the only reliable test used for the diagnosis of heart attack. The test can indicate the presence of a new or old heart attack and a host of other conditions.

STRESS TEST

The ECG done during exercise (stress test) usually helps to confirm the diagnosis of angina and can be used for future reference to detect the progression of the coronary artery disease. The test is very helpful in selecting patients for coronary angioplasty or bypass surgery. Other aspects of the stress test are discussed in Exercise and the Heart.

CHEST X-RAY

A chest X-ray is usually normal in patients with angina but is always abnormal in patients with heart failure, and is often abnormal in those with significant valvular disease, heart muscle disease and congenital heart disease.

NUCLEAR SCANS

The *thallium scan* is useful in selected patients with angina to show the areas of the heart muscle that are poorly perfused with blood. The technique is simple and nonpainful. During an exercise stress test, usually on the treadmill, a known minute amount of radioisotope, thallium-201, is injected into a vein. The thallium reaches the heart and is distributed through the coronary arteries. The areas of the heart muscle that are not receiving adequate blood flow because of blockage of the coronary arteries will receive less thallium, and these areas are assessed by special scanners. Several errors in methods and interpretation limit the usefulness of this test. It is not sufficiently sensitive or specific for coronary heart disease. The test is expensive and time consuming; the information gained is often not sufficiently accurate. The test is much abused by internists and cardiologists who have an interest in nuclear laboratories. Health-care costs can be contained if such tests are limited. These tests should be done only when treatment decisions can be appropriately altered by their results.

Single photon emission computerized tomography (SPECT) uses a new type of scanner plus tomography. The American Heart Association task force indicates that SPECT is not superior or more specific than the simple, planar thallium scan. It is nonetheless more expensive. Positron emission tomography (PET) is an extremely expensive test, fortunately available only in a few research centers. The advantages over SPECT need to be determined by studies to justify the high cost. Nuclear scans give only clues to the presence of cardiac disease and have limited value in making decisions that relate to the choice of treatment for the patient. False positive tests are common. In most instances the cost of these tests is not justifiable. If the ECG is normal it is unlikely that a nuclear scan would be helpful. *If a patient can do nine minutes on an ECG treadmill test using the Bruce Protocol, then a nuclear scan is not expected to add valuable information.*

Another relatively noninvasive test that gives a good estimation of how much blood the heart ejects with each beat (*ejection fraction*) is the gated cardiac scan. With each beat, the normal heart expels at least 50 percent of the blood contained in each ventricle. The percentage ejected is called the ejection fraction, and it is one of the best indicators of the efficiency and strength of heart contraction. The normal ejection fraction is between 50 and 75 percent. The ejection fraction is one of the most important measurements used by the cardiologist to judge the strength or functional capacity of the heart. The ejection fraction is accurately measured during coronary arteriography, and with a similar degree of accuracy, it can be determined with the gated cardiac pool study. In this test a radioisotope, technetium, is injected into an arm vein; the isotope binds to red blood cells and reaches the chambers of the heart. In particular, the left ventricle is well seen with sophisticated scintillation cameras and the data is processed by computer. The force of contraction and the motion of the heart muscle wall is visualized on a video screen. If the muscle is contracting poorly or contracting abnormally, as might be expected with an aneurysm, this can be detected in many cases. This test does not show structure inside the heart. Visualization of structures such as valves inside the heart and *an ejection fraction can be obtained with an echocardiogram, so the echocardiogram is most often used instead of a gated scan.*

Coronary arteriography indications (arteriograms or angiograms) include the following:

- The most important reason to have this test is the presence of angina (see Angina) that interferes with lifestyle to such an extent that it is deemed unacceptable by the patient and the physician. The majority of patients with stable angina are able to live with the occasional occurrence of the fleeting chest discomfort that they know will be precipitated by a particular exertion or emotion. They realize that the pain does not damage the heart muscle and that on stopping the precipitating activity, pain or discomfort disappears immediately or is quickly relieved by a nitroglycerin tablet. Such patients may learn to live with angina from one to 20 years, and nothing else is done. Symptoms can be further improved in many by the use of beta-blockers and in some with the addition of an oral nitrate or calcium blocker. The combination of drugs greatly reduces the occurrence of chest pain. In a few patients with stable angina, pain may occur daily and can interfere with work or lifestyle. Despite the fleeting nature of the pain, the patient may not be satisfied to live with this annoyance and may ask, "What else can be done?" The doctor in many cases may suggest that a coronary arteriogram be done. Thus the doctor-patient relationship is of utmost importance in patients with angina.
- Patients with unstable angina will need arteriography within a few weeks or months after their pain has subsided. The majority of these patients will need to undergo coronary angioplasty or bypass surgery. If surgery is contraindicated because of other medical problems or age, then there is little point to submit the patient to the test.
- There are a few patients in whom the diagnosis of angina is confusing, especially when symptoms or reflux esophagitis

make the diagnosis difficult. Coronary arteriograms may be necessary to unravel the mystery and prevent patients from becoming cardiac cripples.

To re-emphasize, the main reason for having a coronary arteriogram is to show what part of the coronary artery is blocked and to what extent, so as to determine whether the individual is a candidate for coronary angioplasty or coronary artery bypass surgery (see Coronary Artery Bypass Surgery, Figs. 1 and 2). Therefore, we always ensure, first, that the patient is a suitable candidate for surgery, that is, that the angina is severe enough that he or she will need to undergo surgery to relieve the pain, and, second, that there are no medical conditions such as severe bronchitis that may contraindicate surgery.

Coronary arteriography remains the most important method of defining the presence and severity of atherosclerosis of the coronary artery. This test also reveals the size and shape of the left ventricle as well as its ability to contract evenly and forcibly, and problems with valves in the heart. More than one million coronary arteriograms are performed in the United States annually. The procedure is not painful, and depending on the center, the patient is usually admitted the night before, the tests are done the next day, and the patient is discharged later that afternoon. In some institutions, facilities exist for a substantial number of patients to have the test done during the day with discharge several hours later if the condition is satisfactory.

The patient is usually advised not to eat solid food after midnight on the day of the examination. Fluids are allowed up to one hour prior to the procedure. The patient is sedated with 5 mg of diazepam (Valium) given orally, and a specially made catheter is introduced either into the right arm artery (brachial artery) under local anesthesia or the artery in the groin (femoral artery). A small opening is made in the artery and a pigtail-like catheter is introduced and passed under X-ray guidance to the aorta and finally to the area where the aorta leaves the heart. At this point, the coronary arteries usually branch from the aorta, and the catheter is directed into the left and then the right coronary artery (see Fig. 2). A dye is injected and can be visualized by means of several X-rays taken in different planes. The X-rays will show the heart and arteries, the normal arteries or ones with blockage by plaques of atheroma similar to those depicted in Figure 1. Any blockage in the coronary artery is clearly visualized. Coronary arteriography is a relatively safe procedure in experienced hands when done in well-equipped laboratories. Mortality is less than 0.05 percent and minor complications are rare.

Because the procedure is not without complications, the test must be justifiable and the patient must be aware of the risks attached. Patients are usually very keen to have the procedure since they understand it is the only way to know, without doubt, the extent and severity of the coronary obstruction. As well, angioplasty or surgery cannot be done without first visually examining the vessels (an X-ray movie is made and can be replayed during surgery to show the blockages).

ECHOCARDIOGRAM

The echocardiogram is a painless, noninvasive diagnostic technique that utilizes ultrasound. It gives the cardiologist a superb, simple, no-risk evaluation of the valves of the heart, the heart muscle, the force contraction of the muscle and the determination of the ejection fraction. The size of each chamber can be measured, and in particular, enlargement of the heart muscle can be easily defined.

Because the muscle contraction can be visualized, echocardiography is used in some patients after an acute heart attack to detect special complications. The test is most useful in patients with pericarditis and to detect water accumulation around the heart (pericardial effusion). The echocardiogram is thus a most useful test.

HOLTER MONITOR

The Holter monitor is utilized to detect abnormal heart rhythms, particularly in patients with coronary heart disease and other types of heart disease. The machine, about the size of this book, records a continuous electrocardiogram for 24 hours. The instrument is strapped to the waist, and the patient returns home and carries on all normal activities, as well as sleep. After 24 hours, the machine is returned to the doctor's office or hospital. The tape is played and a recording is made. The doctor studies the tracings and determines the number of premature beats (extra beats) that occurred during this period and whether the abnormal beats require treatment. The test is requested when patients complain of palpitations with or without fainting, or when the doctor detects premature beats on listening with the stethoscope or sees such disturbances of rhythm on the electrocardiogram or during a stress test.

TECHNIQUE FOR CARDIAC CATHETERIZATION CORONARY ARTERIOGRAPHY

The procedure is carried out in a cardiac catheterization laboratory under sterile conditions. The most common sites for inserting the wire or hollow plastic catheter are in the femoral artery located in the groin or the artery in the arm at the elbow. These sites are preferred because the blood vessels are large and close to the skin surface.

The pulsation of the artery is easily felt and the skin is anesthetized with a local injection of anesthetic. When the skin is frozen and painless, a needle followed by thin wires is used to introduce the catheter into the artery. The catheter is then guided into the aorta and then into the cavity of the left ventricle. The catheter position is visualized at all times with the aid of an X-ray fluoroscope, which shows the catheter on a screen. This procedure is called cardiac catheterization. The same technique is utilized for performing coronary arteriography (angiograms) or for studying the heart valves and pressures inside the heart chambers.

For coronary angioplasty, a specialized catheter is used. It has a double lumen and a small inflatable balloon at the tip (see Fig. 6). The length of the balloon is about 2.5 cm and the inflated diameter is 2 to 4 mm. The catheter is guided into the appropriate coronary artery to the obstruction previously visualized by coronary arteriography. During coronary arteriography, dye that looks white on X-ray film (radio-opaque) is injected into a catheter positioned selectively in the right and the left coronary arteries.

All patients undergoing coronary angioplasty or coronary artery bypass surgery must have coronary arteriography to show the cardiologist or surgeon the exact site of blockage by a plaque of atheroma (see Fig. 1). Arteriography can be done several hours or a few weeks prior to angioplasty, surgery or other procedures.

Thyroid Heart Disease

High Thyroid (Hyperthyroidism)

The thyroid gland in the neck may suddenly become overactive and secrete excessive amounts of the hormone thyroxine. This situation is not uncommon between age 20 and 50, but can occur later in life. Excessive thyroxine causes increased metabolism of all tissues, therefore weight loss commonly occurs, despite a good appetite. Individuals feel nervous, anxious, irritable and have intolerance to heat. The heart beats faster, the pulse rate may be 110 to 130 beats per minute at rest. Occasionally, abnormal heart rhythms occur, particularly a condition called atrial fibrillation. The fast heart rate may require control with a beta-blocker until treatment with radioactive iodine causes destruction of the gland. Surgery is now rarely used.

Low Thyroid (Hypothyroidism)

This problem is common in the elderly but can occasionally affect individuals age 20 to 60. Lack of the hormone thyroxine causes weight gain, constipation, lethargy, sleepiness, a hoarse voice, dry, puffy, skin and intolerance to cold. Hypothyroidism or myxedema causes a slow pulse rate. The heart may be affected rarely.

Patients who have hyperthyroidism treated with radioactive iodine or surgery become hypothyroid after 10 to 20 years, and require treatment. Thus, hypothyroidism is a common condition in the elderly. The disease can exist for many years before it is recognized by patients or detected by physicians. A simple blood test, sensitive TSH, rapidly and accurately identifies patients who have hypothyroidism and hyperthyroidism. Patients with hypothyroidism require replacement therapy with thyroxine, usually a dosage of .05 to .2 mg daily (50 to 200 micrograms).

TRIGLYCERIDES

Carbohydrates are converted in the body to glucose and triglycerides, and most overweight individuals have an increase in blood triglyceride levels. Excess alcohol consumption and diabetes are well-known causes of marked elevations in triglycerides. Fortunately, weight reduction, cessation of alcohol, and exercise rapidly decrease blood triglycerides. Normal values are 50 to 300 mg/dL (3 mmol), but values up to 400 mg should cause no panic and do not require expensive repeat testing. Elevations of 400 to 2,000 mg are commonly due to obesity or alcohol, and rarely, a genetic defect.

If your triglycerides are elevated, the first step is to repeat the estimation a few months later; no food or drink except water should be taken for 14 hours prior to the test, otherwise a false elevation will be obtained. If levels remain elevated higher than 300 mg, a weight reduction diet low in carbohydrates and alcohol along with regular moderate exercise will cause a 20 to 33 percent decrease over a few months. Hypertriglyceridemia (high triglyceride blood level), unlike high blood cholesterol, responds extremely well to diet or drugs. In a few patients, if levels remain above 500 mg after six months of nondrug therapy, your doctor may prescribe gemfibrozil (Lopid), 600 mg twice daily, or Lipidil micro once daily. These drugs markedly decrease triglycerides with mild lowering of cholesterol and cause a significant increase in HDL ("good") cholesterol.

Hypertriglyceridemia is not considered a significant risk factor for the development of coronary heart disease. When a triglyceride level greater than 500 mg is combined with an elevation of LDL cholesterol and an HDL cholesterol level of less than 30 mg (.7 mmol), the situation warrants treatment with diet and an appropriate drug.

TYPE A BEHAVIOR

Type A individuals have an impatient, time-conscious, achievement-striving personality, and often seek out a hectic environment that provokes undue stress. Leisure brings a feeling of guilt, since their lives are an everlasting struggle against time, toward achievement and recognition. The Type A individual takes on a project, including simple reading, with a certain violence. Speech is often harsh, explosive or aggressive. When stressed, Type A individuals have been shown to release more adrenaline and noradrenaline and to have a greater rise in blood pressure than Type Bs. Type B people are easygoing, able to relax, and rarely carry work home or set deadlines. Most of us are mixtures of Type A and B. It is difficult for a Type A person to change, but with expert assistance, modification of lifestyle is possible.

Friedman and Rosenman have defined and established the concept of the Type A behavior pattern. They emphasized that if you have Type A behavior, you have an increased risk of coronary heart disease. Several studies have confirmed that a relationship exists between Type A behavior and risk of coronary heart disease. This occurs in both men and women independent of high blood cholesterol, hypertension and smoking. The National Heart Lung Blood Institute has accepted the evidence regarding Type A behavior and increased risk of coronary heart disease.

The question of Type A behavior and increased risk of coronary heart disease remains controversial, however. The large Multiple Risk Factor Intervention Study and a small British study did not show any relationship. A study reported in the *New England Journal of Medicine* in March 1985 found no relationship between Type A behavior and mortality from coronary heart disease in patients who had had a heart attack and were followed for three years. Commencing two weeks after their heart attack, 510 patients were followed. At the end of three years, death rate was not related to behavior, whether Type A or Type B. The mean Type A score did not differ significantly from the score of those who survived.

Note that we did not discuss Type A behavior under the section on stress, since these two issues represent two independent factors.

VALVE DISEASES

The valves of the heart (see Fig. 19) are like automatic doors, which open when people want to pass through and stay shut when not in use. When blood must be expelled from the left ventricle into the aorta, the aortic valve, the main valve, opens. The texture of valves is as smooth as silk, thus blood particles and bacteria do not adhere to them. Valves may be the site of disease, however.

MURMURS

When affected by disease, the soft heart valve tissue gets rough, thick, swollen and hard, and as blood rushes through the obstructing or damaged valves, turbulence occurs. The turbulence sets up vibrations that are louder than normal and can be heard easily with a stethoscope. The sound heard by the stethoscope is called a murmur. The loudness of the murmur depends on the velocity of blood flow, the amount of blood passing across the deformed valve and the turbulence that occurs. A cardiologist, using the simple stethoscope and without expensive tests, can tell if a murmur is significant. An echocardiogram confirms this observation but is often unnecessary if the doctor is well trained in the use of a stethoscope. Abuse of this expensive test is common practice. The echocardiogram may display murmurs that are not significant and may create a worry for individuals.

Murmurs are most commonly systolic in time; that is, they occur during the contraction of the ventricles. Many systolic murmurs are not significant in that they do not disturb the function of the heart. Murmurs that occur when the ventricles are relaxed, that is, during diastole, are termed diastolic murmurs and are always of significance (see Murmurs).

Over a period of five to 50 years, significant murmurs increase the work of the heart muscle and cause it to enlarge. The muscle finally becomes weak and heart failure occurs. When heart failure occurs, it is not the end of the life (see Heart Failure).

CAUSES OF VALVE DISEASE

Damage to heart valves is caused by:

- Rheumatic fever.
- Infections, in particular, bacterial endocarditis and syphilis; fortunately, viral infection, though extremely common, is not known to cause valve disease.
- Mitral valve prolapse.

STRUCTURE OF THE HEART

FIGURE 19

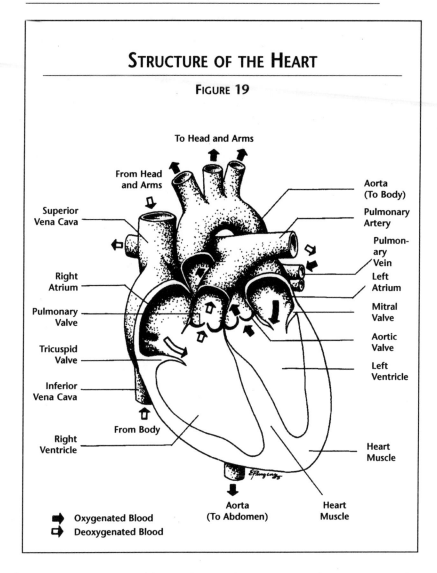

Oxygenated Blood
Deoxygenated Blood

- Rare congenital heart disease (see Congenital Heart Disease).
- Others: coronary heart disease, cardiomyopathy, and degenerative diseases due to age changes, such as calcific aortic sclerosis.

CONSEQUENCES OF VALVE DISEASE

- A murmur is produced and is easily heard by the doctor (see Murmurs).

- Infections may occur on the valve; this is called bacterial endocarditis.
- Complications due to blockage of the valve (stenosis) or backward leak (regurgitation) of blood may cause severe shortness of breath, and balloon valvuloplasty or surgery may be required in a few cases.
- Roughness of the valve may also extend into the chamber of the left atrium and set up electrical discharges. Thus premature beats and palpitations including paroxysmal atrial tachycardia (PAT) and atrial fibrillation may occur.

The major symptoms of serious valve disease are increasing shortness of breath on mild exertion and on lying flat, cough and occasionally blood-tinged sputum (hemoptysis). Finally, signs of heart failure occur, and these include severe shortness of breath, edema of the legs and water in and around the lungs (see Heart Failure).

RHEUMATIC FEVER

Damage to heart valves commonly occurs during an attack of rheumatic fever. Rheumatic fever is most common between the ages of five and 25 and occurs in susceptible individuals after a streptococcal sore throat. The streptococcus bacterium sets up an allergic-like reaction on the valves and in the joints. There is usually fever, joint pains and murmurs over the swollen heart valves, and a blood test to show a reaction to the streptococcus usually confirms the diagnosis.

Fortunately, sore throats caused by the particular type of streptococcus have become much less common and the disease is disappearing from North America. The disease persists and is common in third-world countries.

Not all individuals who get rheumatic fever develop damage to the heart valves. Those who have severe fever with severe joint pains lasting several months may never get valve damage. The opposite is most likely to occur: it appears that when rheumatic fever *"licks the joints it spares the heart."* More than 40 percent of patients may not recall having had an illness with fever and joint pains yet their valves may be affected by minor streptococcal infection.

The mitral valve is commonly affected, followed by the aortic valve, causing conditions called mitral stenosis and regurgitation or aortic stenosis and regurgitation. Other valves rarely get damaged by rheumatic fever or degenerative disease.

Prevention of Rheumatic Fever

Rheumatic fever tends to recur in the same individual because of a particular predisposition. In order to prevent recurrence, the following is advised: If rheumatic fever was properly documented, but there is no evidence of significant valve damage, penicillin is usually given for a minimum of five years or to age 20, whichever is longest. If the heart valve was damaged, penicillin is given for a minimum of 10 years or to age 40, whichever is the longest. Depending on the state or country, and the prevalence of beta-hemolytic streptococci and rheumatic fever, some physicians continue treatment beyond age 40. The dose of antibiotic is usually one of the following:

1. Penicillin-V, 250 mg twice daily. If the patient is allergic to penicillin, sulfadiazine is as effective — 1 g once daily for adults and 0.5 g daily for patients weighing less than 60 pounds.
2. 1.2 million units of benzathine penicillin G intramuscularly, given monthly.

MITRAL STENOSIS

The silky, soft leaflets of the mitral valve become thickened, rough and hard, and over a few years the orifice of the valve becomes tight. Blood in the left atrium has difficulty getting through the mitral valve to reach the left ventricle (see Fig. 19). When the orifice is severely narrowed, blood backs up into the lung and causes severe shortness of breath and heart failure.

The treatment of severe mitral stenosis is by balloon valvuloplasty or surgery, which is necessary if severe shortness of breath is present and persistent.

Valvuloplasty involves passing a catheter and guidewire through the artery from the groin into the heart to the tight valve, which is then snapped open with a balloon-tipped catheter. The procedure is highly successful and is suitable for more than 75 percent of patients. If this procedure cannot be done, surgery is recommended.

Surgery is relatively simple and safe; the valve is opened with a finger-like or a special metal dilator. In a few cases the valve may also have a leaking problem and must be replaced by a prosthesis. The results of surgery are excellent but reserved for patients with severe symptoms. Many patients can live five to 30 years with mild to moderate symptoms before they become serious enough to warrant valvuloplasty or surgery. Complications are rare except when atrial fibrillation occurs. Digoxin and an anticoagulant are then required.

MITRAL REGURGITATION

The valve may be diseased in such a manner that it does not close tightly during contraction of the left ventricle. When the mitral valve is not shut tight, blood leaks or regurgitates from the ventricle back into the left atrium, thus the leaking valve is called mitral regurgitation. These patients tolerate the leak for many years and, in a few, the left ventricle as well as the left atrium can become enlarged; shortness of breath occurs and surgery to replace the valve may be necessary. Patients can tolerate the lesions for five to 30 years depending on their degree. In some patients heart failure occurs, and they require drug treatment and surgery; surgery should be done before heart failure develops. The timing for surgery is very difficult.

AORTIC STENOSIS

Aortic stenosis is usually due to previous rheumatic fever or calcification in the elderly; in young patients, a congenital bicuspid valve may become calcified, hardened and narrowed over 10 to 50 years. In aortic stenosis, the aortic valve (see Fig. 19) is tight and obstructs the flow of blood from the left ventricle into the aorta; less blood reaches the head. Symptoms such as dizziness, fainting, shortness of breath and chest pain may occur. The left ventricle tries to overcome the obstruction by pumping more forcefully, and over years, the muscle enlarges and finally fails. A few cases may require surgery; severe shortness of breath, chest pains, fainting spells, enlargement of the left ventricle or heart failure are indications for surgery.

The diseased valve is removed and an aortic valve prosthesis is usually inserted. This is extensive surgery and is done only when justifiable. Any patient over age 45 may have concomitant coronary heart disease and may require valve replacement as well as coronary artery bypass graft.

Aortic Regurgitation

In this condition, the aortic valve remains widely open when it should be tightly closed, therefore blood regurgitates or leaks from the aorta backward into the left ventricle (see Fig. 19). The left ventricle has more work to do and over several years dilates and enlarges. Surgery is not often required because the left ventricle copes with the extra work for many years and drugs such as captopril (an ACE inhibitor) can prevent progression of the leak. Leaking valves impose less work on the heart than obstructed valves. When heart failure occurs due to a leaking valve, digoxin and diuretics are helpful as well as vasodilators such as captopril and enalapril. Surgery is required to replace the valve before heart failure occurs. The timing for surgery can be very difficult to estimate. Surgical intervention is not without risks.

To re-emphasize, a tight valve is medically called a stenosis, thus the terms "mitral stenosis" and "aortic stenosis." A leaky valve indicates regurgitation of blood, and the two common lesions are mitral regurgitation and aortic regurgitation. The pulmonary and tricuspid valves are rarely affected except when due to congenital heart disease or infection caused by endocarditis, particularly in drug addicts.

Prosthetic heart valve surgery is a major undertaking and careful assessment by a cardiology team is necessary. Post surgery, the patient may need to take anticoagulants to prevent clotting on the valve. Warfarin is given if a mechanical valve is used or if atrial fibrillation is present. A bioprosthesis is advised in patients over age 65, and no blood thinners are required with these valves.

Case History

At age 29 Mrs. J. B. started having a cough with shortness of breath, mainly on climbing stairs. Over the next few weeks, symptoms occurred at night in bed. Cough, shortness of breath, and wheezing became worse over the next month, and her family doctor prescribed cough medicines. About one month later there was no improvement. At night she would have difficulty breathing and would have to sit up for a half to one hour to get some relief. The second visit to the doctor resulted in a 12-day course of antibiotics and another cough medicine to clear the chest infection or congestion in the lungs.

Several weeks later she was no better; more cough medicine was prescribed along with an inhaler to try and relieve her bronchial spasms. There was no fever or chills. At this stage she had difficulty doing her housework and climbing stairs, chiefly because of shortness of breath and cough. She noted that her sputum was tinged with blood at times. She smoked 20 to 30 cigarettes per day and was advised to give this up since she had bronchitis and congestion.

At this stage she was referred to the cardiologist. She had the typical heart sounds and murmur of mitral stenosis. The valve was extremely tight, and blood was backing up, congesting and flooding the lungs. She was admitted to the hospital that day. Her shortness of breath was 50 percent relieved by the diuretic furosemide and she was able to sleep. Her blood-tinged sputum disappeared over the next few days, and three weeks later she had heart catheterization. Cardiac surgery was performed the next month, the valve was opened, and 20 years later she remains healthy and able to do her housework and exercises. The lesson here is that a tight valve (mitral stenosis) and heart failure can mimic other causes of lung congestion and can produce symptoms that resemble asthma and acute bronchitis.

CALCIFIC AORTIC SCLEROSIS

The aortic valve may become calcified and hardened (sclerosed), especially during ages 60 to 80, and the doctor may hear the loud murmur with a stethoscope. Fortunately, the deposits of calcium do not cause significant obstruction to the blood flow. Thus this calcific valve rarely becomes tight enough to cause symptoms, and tests are rarely required. Surgery may be necessary in one out of 10,000 cases. More than 33 percent of individuals over age 70 have a murmur over the aortic valve due to calcific aortic sclerosis.

MITRAL VALVE PROLAPSE

This is a common disease. The mitral valve leaflets become stretched and floppy with redundant folds. The valve is damaged by a degenerative myxomatous process. Using a stethoscope, the doctor hears the valves flapping like a sail in a crisp wind. The noise heard is typical and is called a click and murmur. The click can be similar to a loud tick of a clock or at times it is a musical sound. The condition is somewhat more common in females, and about five percent of individuals over age 25 have this click and murmur, which is produced by the mitral valve and termed mitral valve prolapse. Middle-aged men, however, develop a more complicated valve disturbance.

The condition is benign: less than one in every 100 cases may have a problem. But many people become anxious and nervous about the problem exaggerated by physicians. Panic attacks may occur. A few individuals may have palpitations consisting chiefly of premature beats that rarely cause fainting spells. Beta-blockers are very useful in this condition to relieve bothersome palpitations and faint-like episodes. Chest pain occurs in a few but the condition is not related to coronary heart disease and there is no relation between the disease and heart attacks. In less than one in 1,000 cases, the valve leaflet may weaken or get a redundant fold and cause regurgitation of blood; in such patients mild and sometimes severe mitral regurgitation may occur. In a few surgical repair or valve replacement may be required. In the Western world, severe mitral prolapse is the commonest reason for repair or replacement of the mitral valve in men and women. In third-world countries, rheumatic fever remains the common cause for replacement.

Infection of the valve, causing bacterial endocarditis and further damage, may occur, particularly if a murmur is present. Thus, prophylaxis with antibiotics is advisable before dental work and surgical procedures; otherwise the patient, who can live to 90, may have an abrupt shortening of life.

BACTERIAL ENDOCARDITIS

Valves previously affected by rheumatic fever are thick, rough and swollen. Other causes of deformity of the heart valves have been discussed. Bacteria that gain entry into the bloodstream on their way through the heart may attach to the roughened valve surface and set up an area of infection. The bacteria may grow to form an "abscess" on the valve. The abscess resembles a clump of moss that swings and sways on the valve leaflet as it opens and closes. Infection of the heart valves is called endocarditis. Usually the infection is by bacteria, thus the term bacterial endocarditis.

In susceptible individuals, bacterial endocarditis can begin weeks or months after simple manipulations such as scaling and cleaning of teeth, other dental work, and surgery in areas of the body where infection may gain access. Patients who have mild heart valve lesions but can normally live a normal life to age 90 may have their lives suddenly shortened by this infection.

Prevention of Endocarditis

The American Heart Association recommendations for preventing bacterial endocarditis are as follows:

- Patients with valvular heart disease must be given antibiotics a half to one hour prior to all dental or surgical procedures and six hours later. The antibiotic is given orally for dental work done under local anesthetic. The antibiotic is given intravenously for patients with prosthetic valves, patients with highest risk of developing endocarditis, or patients who are having a general anesthetic. All dental procedures that are likely to result in gingival bleeding such as extractions, root canal, scaling and cleaning, and surgery in the oral cavity, biopsies and many surgical operations and tests such as cystoscopy require antibiotic coverage to prevent endocarditis.
- Oral antibiotic therapy is given when a local anesthetic is used: Amoxicillin, 3 g, one hour prior to and 1.5 g after the procedure. Patients allergic to penicillin usually receive clindamycin, two 150-mg capsules one hour prior to and six hours after the procedure. This regimen is convenient and is not as difficult as taking nine capsules of amoxicillin.

  For surgery on the intestine or the genital or urinary systems, other antibiotics are required intravenously. You must warn the doctor in the hospital or your dentist that you have a heart valve disease and require antibiotics prophylactically.

A British Society Working Party recommendation for endocarditis prevention during dental procedures recommends the following: When dental work is done under local anesthetic, if there is no allergy to penicillin, 3 g of amoxicillin are taken orally in the presence of a dentist (1.5 g to children) one hour before the operation. If the surgery is done under general anesthetic for dental work and the patient is not allergic to penicillin, 1 g of amoxicillin is given intramuscularly or intravenously followed by 0.5 g orally six hours later.

Carious teeth and dental work can maim individuals with heart valve defects. The heart valve defect may be a very mild one of very little significance causing no symptoms and yet can become infected. Individuals who have heart murmurs or valve disorders should receive antibiotic coverage to prevent endocarditis.

CASE HISTORY I

Mrs. S., age 69, had a fever of 100 to 104°F with chills and weakness over a period of 14 months. She had attended several clinics and physicians including one period of hospitalization. She was previously quite well and was not known to have heart disease. She had six children; they were alive and healthy, and it was a surprise to them that their previously healthy mother was now bedridden. She was not short of breath and there was no cough. The diagnosis was obvious. The woman had a soft systolic murmur at the apex of the heart and typical swelling of the fingertips near the nail bed called finger clubbing. Clubbing is a hallmark of bacterial endocarditis. On questioning, she admitted that 14 months previously she had had all her teeth removed. She was treated with a combination of penicillin and streptomycin for a period of six weeks and she made an uneventful recovery; 10 years later she was alive and well.

CASE HISTORY II

One unfortunate morning L.H., a 29-year-old female who was known to have a soft heart murmur, was walking to the bathroom and fell to the floor. Her left arm felt weak and her speech was slurred. She was rushed to the hospital, and after three days she made a complete recovery and was discharged.

Three weeks later she had the typical features of finger clubbing, murmur and fever and was admitted to the hospital. She had a temperature of 100 to 102°F. Her blood was taken and cultured and grew a bacteria called streptococcus viridans; this is the most common cause of bacterial endocarditis. She was treated with penicillin and streptomycin for six weeks and made a good recovery. Her previous mild mitral valve regurgitation became moderate. Some 25 years later, she is able to do her usual work, exercises and enjoys life with minimal restrictions. She realizes that surgery may become necessary sometime in the future. You must note how long she has gone without a valve replacement; we trust that this information would allay your anxiety.

We must emphasize that apart from infection of previously damaged heart valves as well as prosthetic valves, normal valves can become damaged. Fortunately this occurs extremely rarely and mainly in drug addicts. The syringe and needles may be contaminated, and germs introduced into the bloodstream can infect valves on the right side of the heart (tricuspid and pulmonary valves). These germs are very actively growing types; thus, they can damage normal valves. The bacteria found in such cases are staphylococcus and pseudomonas.

Preventive medicine has helped to eradicate the dreadful streptococcus not only by the use of antibiotics but also through the relief of overcrowding, the improvement of sanitation and ventilation in disadvantaged socioeconomic groups. Thus, rheumatic fever is now rare in North America but is common in India, Pakistan, Africa, the West Indies and South America.

We can prevent bacterial endocarditis by intelligent use of appropriate antibiotics on the day of dental or other surgery. The rare, very serious valve disorder can be cured surgically in the majority of cases. Heart valve disease is common, but valve surgery has improved in the past 20 years. Patients live a normal life after valve repair or replacement. If a mechanical valve is implanted, blood thinners, anticoagulants, are necessary. In patients over age 69, a bioprosthetic valve is preferred because these function well for 15 to 20 years and no blood thinners are required. Blood thinners are required with both types of implanted valves, however, if atrial fibrillation is present.

VENTRICULAR FIBRILLATION

The heart muscle does not contract but "quivers"; therefore, there is no heartbeat (cardiac arrest). No blood is pumped out of the heart. Death occurs within minutes if the abnormal heart rhythm is not corrected. Ventricular fibrillation requires electrical countershock within three minutes to change this life-threatening rhythm to normal heartbeats. CPR must be instituted immediately to maintain a blood supply to the brain until a defibrillator is available; hopefully within a few minutes. Note that in atrial fibrillation, the atrium fibrillates but the ventricles contract normally although faster than normal; this condition is usually not life-threatening and is easily controlled with the commonly known heart drug digoxin.

WOMEN AND HEART DISEASE

Women incorrectly perceive their risk of cancer of the breast and uterus as much greater than that of heart disease or stroke, and are thus not sufficiently motivated to reduce their risk of heart disease. Yet after age 65, one in three women have some form of cardiovascular disease. More than 350,000 women die of a heart attack and more than 120,000 die of a stroke in the U.S. and Canada each year. The National Center for Health Statistics indicates that for the 12 months ending in August 1994, deaths from cardiovascular disease in the United States were 944,280. Women and men share nearly equally in these horrifying numbers. Mortality figures in Canada are usually 10 percent of the figure quoted for the United States. The 1990 statistics revealed that of all cardiovascular deaths, 56 percent occurred in women and 44 percent in men. This situation is occurring because of the relatively large population of older women. Cardiovascular disease is a much more common cause of death and disability in women than is cancer, pneumonia and AIDS.

Fortunately, most women are protected from the risk of heart attack up to age 48 because of their hormonal status. It is extremely rare for a normal menstruating woman to have a heart attack prior to age 45 except in those who have blood cholesterol at levels greater than 360 mg (9 mmol). The incidence in heart attack in men and women at age 35, 40, 50, 65, 70 and 75 are

100-1, 20-1, 10-1, 5-2, 5-4, 1-1. Because more men age 35 to 65 than women have heart attacks and angina, there are more clinical studies done on men using drugs, coronary bypass surgery and angioplasty. Women believe they are not treated equally by the medical profession particularly in the area of heart disease. *Women are not excluded from studies, they are fortunately not around.* Women believe that there is some bias attached to the treatment of men versus women with heart problems. Some doctors are proclaiming that women with heart disease have different symptoms from men and respond differently to drugs, angioplasty and bypass surgery. This assumption is incorrect. Because not sufficient women age 35 to 65 were available to be included in the studies, information on women and heart disease is deficient. There will still not be sufficient women to be included in studies over the next 20 years. Patients age 71 to 80 are not usually entered into long-term follow-up studies.

Symptoms of a genuine heart attack are not significantly different in women and men. Some women suffer with shortness of breath or nausea instead of pain during a heart attack, but so do a few men. Diagnosis of a heart attack is similar in women and men. The ECG gives the same information in both. It is true that women with so-called atypical chest pain recurring at different times of the day and night have equivocal stress tests, but that is an entirely different situation.

The medical treatment for heart attack is the same for both women and men and the response is the same. It is obvious that there are more 75- to 85-year-old women with heart attacks than men as the population of elderly women is increasing relative to men. At age 75 to 85, women may have a slightly higher risk of bleeding with therapy and doctors will need to reduce the dose of thrombolytic drugs to match the age and weight of women.

Bypass surgery and angioplasty in the elderly carry a greater risk, and the results of angioplasty appear to be less impressive in women. Women who need bypass surgery do just as well as men. Complications of bypass surgery are said to be slightly higher in women. There are no studies done to compare 71- to 81-year-old men and women undergoing bypass surgery and angioplasty. Bypass surgery is done more often in men at a younger age, because this treatment is performed to relieve angina. Angina interferes with lifestyle, particularly the ability to work between age 40 to 60. This is an age at which women are less subjected to disabling angina.

We stated under the section on Hormones that women can decrease their risk of heart attack and stroke by taking estrogens, e.g., Premarin .625 mg or equivalent and aspirin enteric coated 81 mg daily. Asymptomatic women age 55 or greater with a family history of heart attack at age less than 55, a presence of mild hypertension or increase in LDL cholesterol greater than 190 mg/dL (5 mmol/L), with an HDL (good) cholesterol less than 1.2, should be afforded the protection of estrogen and aspirin. Caution is required, however, because the Nurses' Health Study reported in the *New England Journal of Medicine* in June 1995 indicates that the risk of breast cancer was significantly increased among women who were currently using estrogen. Cardiovascular risk and the risk of developing breast cancer should be assessed for each post-menopausal woman prior to the long-term use of estrogen.

Estrogens increase HDL cholesterol and decrease LDL cholesterol. Excellent but expensive cholesterol-lowering agents do not increase HDL cholesterol. All heart drugs and aspirin work equally well in women and men to prevent heart attacks, sudden death and stroke. All blood pressure–lowering medications work equally well in women and men to prevent stroke or heart failure.

STRATEGIES FOR PREVENTION

If you are 50 plus, strategies that may prevent cardiovascular disease include:

- Aspirin, 81 mg daily. An enteric coated 81-mg tablet has been available in the United States for years. It could take five years or more to reach Canada. The widely available non-coated 80-mg tablet is available in Canada. A 325-mg tablet is available but can cause gastric bleeding in some people.
- Discontinuation of smoking.
- Premarin, .3 to .625 mg, if you have had a hysterectomy (if not see discussion under Hormones).
- Premarin, .625 mg and a Progesterone, if you have not had a hysterectomy.
- Maintaining systolic blood pressure at less than 140.
- Maintaining cholesterol at less than 200 mg (5 mmol) or LDL at less than 120 mg (3 mmol) if you have no heart disease and less than 100 mg (2.5 mmol) if you have coronary heart disease.

BIBLIOGRAPHY

Aro A, Kardinaal AFM, Salminen I, et al: Adipose tissue isomeric trans fatty acids and risk of myocardial infarction in nine countries: the EURAMIC study. Lancet 345: 273, 1995.

Aronow WS: Effect of non-nicotine cigarettes and carbon monoxide on angina. Circulation 61:262, 1980.

Aronow WS, Stemmer EA, Zweig S: Carbon monoxide and ventricular fibrillation threshold in normal dogs. Arch Environ Health 34:184, 1979.

Baber NS, Julian DG, Lewis JA, et al.: Beta-blockers after myocardial infarction: have trials changed practice? Br Med J 289:1431, 1984.

Brensike JF, Levy RI, Kelsey SF, et al.: Effects of therapy with cholestyramine on progression of coronary arteriosclerosis: results of the NHLBI Type II Coronary Intervention Study. Circulation 69:313, 1984.

Brown JJ, Lever AF, Robertson TIS, et al.: Salt and hypertension. Lancet II:456, 1984.

Calhoun DA, Oparil S: Hypertensive Crisis since FDR - A partial victory. N Engl J Med 332: 1029, 1995.

Campeau L, Enjarbest M, Lesperance J, et al.: The relation of risk factors to the development of atherosclerosis in saphenous-vein bypass grafts and the progression of disease in the native circulation. A study 10 years after aorto-coronary bypass surgery. N Engl J Med 311:1329, 1984.

Carr AA, Mulligan OF, Sherrill LN: Pindolol versus methyldopa for hypertension: comparison of adverse reactions. Am Heart J 104:479, 1982.

Case RB, Heller SS, Case NB, et al.: Type A behavior and survival after acute myocardial infarction. N Engl J Med 312: 737, 1985.

Castelli WP, Garrison RJ, Dawber TR, et al., The filter cigarette and coronary heart disease: The Framingham Study. Lancet II: 109, 1981.

Cohen IS, Jick H, Cohen SI: Adverse reactions to quinidine in hospitalized patients: findings based on data from the Boston Collaborative Drug Surveillance Program. Prog Cardiovasc Dis 20:151, 1977.

Colditz GA, Hankinson SE, Hunter DJ: The use of estrogens and progestins and the risk of breast cancer in post-menopausal women. N Engl J Med 332:1589, 1995.

Coronary Drug Project Research Group: The Coronary Drug Project. Findings leading to discontinuation of the 2.5 mg/day estrogen group. JAMA 226, 652, 1973.

Cryer PE, Haymond MW, Santiago JV, et al.: Norepinephrine and epinephrine release and adrenergic medication of smoking: associated hemodynamic and metabolic events. N Engl J Med 295:573, 1986.

Davies MJ, Thomas A: Thrombosis and acute coronary-artery lesions in sudden cardiac ischemic death. N Engl J Med 310:1137, 1984.

de Lorgeril M, Renaud S, Mamelle N, et al: Mediterranean alpha-linolenic acid-rich diet in secondary prevention of coronary heart disease. Lancet 343:1454, 1994.

Deanfield JE, Shea M, Kensett M, et al.: Silent myocardial ischemia due to mental stress. Lancet II:1001, 1984.

DeBias DA, Banerjee CM, Birkhead NC, et al.: Effects of carbon monoxide inhalation on ventricular fibrillation. Arch Environ Health 31:38, 1976.

DeWood MA, Spores J, Notske R, et al: Prevalence of total coronary occlusion during the early hours of transmural myocardial infarction. N Engl J Med 303:897, 1980.

Eaker ED, Chesebro JH, Sacks FM, et al: AHA Medical/Scientific Statement Special Report: Cardiovascular disease in women. Circulation 88, 1999, 1993.

Friedman M, Rosenman RH: Type A Behavior and Your Heart. New York, Alfred A. Knopf, 1974.

Furberg CD, Friedewald WT, Eberlein KA (eds): Proceedings of the Workshop on Implications of Recent Beta-Blocker Trials for Post-Myocardial Infarction Patients. Circulation Part II, 67: 1983.

Grier MT, Meyers DG. So much writing, so little science: a review of 37 years of literature on edetate sodium chelation therapy. Ann Pharmacother, 27: 1504, 1993.

Guallar E, Hennekens CG, Sacks FM, et al: A prospective study of plasma fish oil levels and incidence of myocardial infarction in U.S. male physicians. J Am Coll Cardiol 25: 387, 1995.

Haft JI, Fani K: Intravascular platelet aggregation in the heart induced by stress. Circulation 47:353, 1973.

Haft JI, Fani K: Stress and the induction of intravascular platelet aggregation in the heart. Circulation 48:164, 1973.

Harris WS, Connor WE, McMurry MP: The comparative reduction of the plasma lipids and lipoproteins by dietary polyunsaturated fats: salmon oil versus vegetable oil. Metabolism 32:179, 1983.

Isner JM, Sours HE, Pares AL, et al.: Sudden, unexpected death in avid dieters using the liquid-protein-modified-fast diet. Circulation 60:1401, 1979.

Katan MB: Fish and Heart Disease. N Engl J Med 332: 1024, 1995.

Keatinge WR, Coleshaw SRK, Cotter F, et al.: Increase in platelet and red cell counts, blood viscosity, and arterial pressure during mild surface cooling: factors in mortality from coronary and cerebral thrombosis in winter. Br Med J 289:1405, 1984.

Khan MG: Cardiac and Pulmonary Management. Philadelphia, Lea & Febiger, 1993.

Khan MG: Cardiac Drug Therapy, 4th edition. London, WB Saunders, 1995.

Lakka TA, Venalainen JM, Rauramaa R, et al: Relation of leisure-time physical activity and cardiorespiratory fitness to the risk of acute myocardial infarction in men. N Engl J Med 330: 1549, 1994.

Landau C, Lange RA, Hillis D, et al: Percutaneous Transluminal coronary angioplasty. N Engl J Med 330:981, 1994.

Lewis HD, Davis JW, Archibald DG, et al: Protective effects of aspirin against acute myocardial infarction and death in men with unstable angina: results of a Veterans Administration Cooperative Study. N Engl J Med 309:396, 1983.

McKeigue P. Trans fatty acids and coronary heart disease: weighing the evidence against hardened fat. Lancet 345: 269, 1995.

Meydani M: Vitamin E. Lancet 345: 170, 1995.

Milvey P, Siegel AJ: Physical activity levels and altered mortality from coronary heart disease with an emphasis on marathon running: A critical review. Cardiovasc Rev 2:233, 1981.

Morris JN, Hagan A, Patterson DC, et al.: Incidence and prediction of ischemic heart disease in London busmen. Lancet II:553, 1966.

Multiple Risk Factor Intervention Trial Research Group: Multiple risk factor intervention trial: risk factor changes and mortality results. JAMA 248:1465, 1982.

Norwegian Multicenter Study Group: Timolol-induced reduction in mortality and reinfarction in patients surviving acute myocardial infarction, N Engl J Med 304:801, 1981.

O'Laughlin MP, Mullins CE: Catheterization cures of congenital heart disease. Cardiol Rev 1:2, 97, 1993.

Oliver MF, MAAS Investigators: Effect of simvastatin on coronary atheroma: the Multicentre Anti-Atheroma Study. Lancet 344: 633, 1994.

Paffenbarger RS Jr, Hale WE: Work activity and coronary heart mortality. N Engl J Med 292:545, 1975.

Paffenbarger RS Jr, Wing AL, Hyde RT; Physical activity as an index of heart attack risk in college allumni. Am J Epidemiol 108:161, 1978.

Review Panel on Coronary-Prone Behavior and Coronary Heart Disease. Coronary-prone behavior and coronary heart disease. A critical review. Circulation 63:1199, 1981.

Robert TL, Wood DA, Riemersma RA et al: Trans isomers of oleic and linoleic acids in adipose tissue and sudden cardiac death. Lancet 345: 278, 1995.

Scandinavian Simvastatin Survivial Study Group: Randomized trial of cholesterol lowering in 4444 patients with coronary heart disease: the Scandinavian Simvastatin Survival Study (4S). Lancet 344: 1383, 1994. Criqui MH, Ringel BL: Does diet or alcohol explain the French paradox?. Lancet 344, 1719, 1994.

Serruys PW, de Jaegere P, Kiemeneij F, et al: A comparison of balloon-expandable-stent implantation with balloon angioplasty in patients with coronary artery disease. N Engl J Med 331:489, 1994.

Siscovick DS, Weiss NS, Fletcher RH, et al.: The incidence of primary cardiac arrest during vigorous exercise. N Engl J Med 311:874, 1984.

Spence JD: Effects of antihypertensive agents on blood velocity: implications for atherogenesis. Can Med Assoc J 127:721, 1982.

The Lipid Research Clinics Program: The Lipid Research Clinics Coronary Primary Prevention Trial Results: I. The relationship of reduction in incidence of coronary heart disease to cholesterol lowering. JAMA 251:365, 1984.

The Writing Group for the (PEPI) Trial: Effects of estrogen or estrogen/progestin regimens on heart disease risk factors in postmenopausal women. JAMA 273: 199, 1995.

Thompson PD, Funk EJ, Carleton RA, et al.: incidence of death during jogging in Rhode Island from 1975 through 1980. JAMA 247:2535, 1982.

Thompson PD, Stern WP, Williams P, et al.: Death during jogging or running: study of 18 cases. JAMA 242:1265, 1979.

van Rij AM, Solomon C, Packer SGK, et al. Chelation therapy for intermittent claudication: a double-blind, randomized controlled trial. Circulation 90:1194, 19″4.

Virag R, Bouilly P, Frydman D: Is impotence an arterial disorder. Lancet I:181, 1985.

Wald NJ, Howard S, Smith PG, et al.: Association between atherosclerotic distress and carboxyhemoglobin levels in tobacco smokers. Br Med J I:761, 1973.

Waller BF, Roberts WC: Sudden death while running in conditioned runners aged 40 years or over. Am J Cardiol 45:1292, 1980.

Wood AJ. Drug Therapy: Hormonal treatment of postmenopausal women. N Engl J Med 330: 1062, 1994.

GLOSSARY

Aneurysm: A severe weakening of the wall of an artery or heart muscle, leading to ballooning of the wall of the vessel or heart.

Angina pectoris: Chest pain due to severe but temporary lack of blood and oxygen to a part of the heart muscle.

Aorta: Main artery arising from the heart; the branches of the aorta take blood to all parts of the body.

Arrhythmia: General term for an irregularity or rapidity of the heartbeat.

Arteriosclerosis: Loss of elasticity and hardening of arteries due to all causes such as age change, deposits of calcium or deposits of atheroma.

Artery: Blood vessels that carry blood away from the heart to organs, tissues and cells throughout the body, as opposed to veins, which carry blood from the tissues back to the heart.

Atheroma: A hardened plaque in the wall of an artery: the plaque is filled with cholesterol, calcium and other substances. The plaque of atheroma hardens the artery, hence the term "atherosclerosis" (sclerosis — hardening).

Atrium: One of two upper chambers of the heart.

Calorie: A unit of energy; one calorie represents the amount of heat required to raise the temperature of one kilogram of water one degree Celsius. The energy present in foods is measured in calories.

Cardiac arrest: Cessation of the heartbeat.

Cardiac catheterization: A cardiac catheter is inserted through a vein or artery and pushed and propelled to reach inside the heart. The progress of the catheter is watched on a fluoroscope.

Catheter: A flexible tube that can be inserted into body organs to achieve drainage, treatment, or diagnosis.

Cholesterol: A lipid, or fat-like substance, made by animal cells.

Coronary thrombosis: A blood clot in a coronary artery, blocking blood flow to a part of the heart muscle. Also called a heart attack or myocardial infarction.

Embolism, embolus: A blood clot or clump of platelets that forms in an artery, a vein or the heart and breaks off and is carried by the circulating blood, finally lodging and blocking the artery that supplies an organ with blood. For example, a pulmonary embolism is an embolus blocking an artery in the lung.

Hemoglobin: Heme — "iron," globin — "protein"; an iron-protein substance present in red blood cells that carries oxygen to the cells of the body.

Infarct or infarction: An area of cells that die as a result of blockage of an artery that brings blood to these cells.

Ischemia: Temporary lack of blood and oxygen to an area of cells (e.g., heart muscle), usually due to severe obstruction of the artery supplying blood to this area of cells. Thus the term "ischemic heart disease" is synonymous with coronary artery disease or coronary heart disease.

Murmur: A noise or extra sound heard between normal heartbeats. The doctor hears the sound with a stethoscope.

Myocardial infarction (infarct): Death of an area of heart muscle due to blockage of a coronary artery by blood clot and atheroma; medical term for a heart attack.

Myocardium: The heart muscle.

Pericarditis: Inflammation of the pericardium or sac surrounding the heart; this is not a heart attack.

Pericardium: The thin, tough membrane or sac that surrounds the heart.

Platelets: Very small disc-like particles that circulate in the blood and initiate the formation of blood clots. Platelets clump and form little plugs, thus stopping bleeding.

Stroke: Damage of part of the brain due to blockage or rupture of an artery in the brain, which leads to weakness or paralysis of limbs with or without disturbances of speech or consciousness. A stroke or cerebrovascular accident is not a form of heart attack.

Ventricle: One of the two lower chambers of the heart.

Ventricular fibrillation: The heart muscle does not contract but "quivers"; therefore, there is no heartbeat (cardiac arrest). No blood is pumped out of the heart. Death occurs within minutes if the abnormal heart rhythm is not corrected. Note that in atrial fibrillation, the atrium fibrillates but the ventricles contract normally although faster than normal; this condition is usually not life-threatening and is easily controlled with the commonly known heart drug digoxin.

Appendix A

GENERIC	PHARMACEUTICAL TRADE NAME

BLOOD PRESSURE PILLS

Beta-Blockers

Acebutolol	Monitan, Sectral
Atenolol	Tenormin
Labetalol	Normodyne, Trandate
Metoprolol	Betaloc, Lopressor, Toprol XL
Nadolol	Corgard
Pindolol	Visken
Propranolol	Inderal, Inderal LA
Timolol	Blocadren, Betim
Sotalol	Sotacor

Diuretics

Thiazides

Chlorothiazide	Diuril, Saluric
Hydrochlorothiazide	HydroDiuril, Esidrix, Oretic, Direma
Bendrofluazide	Aprinox, Berkozide, Centyl, Neo-Naclex
Metolazone	Zaroxolyn, Metenix

Strong diuretics

Furosemide, frusemide	Lasix, Dryptal
Bumetanide	Burinex, Bumex
Ethacrynic acid	Edecrin
Torsemide	Demadex

Diuretics that retain potassium
Amiloride	Midamor
Spironolactone	Aldactone
Triamterene	Dyrenium, Dytac

*Thiazide combined with
potassium-retaining diuretic*
Nongeneric names	Aldactazide
	Dyazide
	Moduretic, Moduret

Vasodilators (dilate arteries)
ACE Inhibitors
Benazepril	Lotensin
Captopril	Capoten
Cilazapril	Inhibace
Enalapril	Vasotec
Fosinopril	Monopril
Lisinopril	Prinivil, Zestril
Perindopril	Coversyl
Quinapril	Accupril
Ramipril	Altace

Angiotensin II Receptor Blocker
Losartan	Cozzar
Losartan plus hydrochlorothiazide	Hyzzar

Calcium Antagonists
Amlodipine	Norvasc
Nifedipine	Adalat XL, Procardia XL
Diltiazem	Cardizem CD
Felodipine	Plendil, Renedil
Verapamil	Isoptin

Other Antihypertensives
Clonidine	Catapres
Guanabenz	Wytensin
Methyldopa	Aldomet, Dopamet
Reserpine	Abicol, Decaserpyl, Raudixin, Serpasil

DRUGS USED FOR ANGINA

Nitrates

Nitroglycerin (sublingual)	Nitrostat, Nitro–Bid, Nitrolingual Spray
Isosorbide dinitrate	Coronex, Isordil, Sorbitrate, others
Isosorbide mononitrate	Imdur Ismo

Beta-Blockers. See above.

Calcium Antagonists

Diltiazem	Anginyl, Cardizem, Cardizem CD
Nifedipine	Adalat XL, Procardia XL
Verapamil	Calan, Cordilox, Isoptin, Isoptin SR, Isoptino

DRUGS FOR HEART FAILURE

Digoxin	Lanoxin, others
Furosemide and other diuretics. See above.	
ACE Inhibitors such as captopril and enalapril. See above.	

DRUGS FOR ABNORMAL HEART RHYTHMS (ARRHYTHMIAS)

Amiodarone	Cordarone, Cordarone X
Beta-Blockers. See above.	
Digoxin	Lanoxin
Disopyramide	Norpace, Rythmodan
Mexiletine	Mexitil
Procainamide	Pronestyl
Quinidine	Cardioquin, Quinidex Quinate, Biquin, Durules
Sotalol	Sotacor

DRUGS THAT AFFECT BLOOD CLOTTING

Blood Thinners: Anticoagulants

Warfarin	Coumadin, Warfilone, Marevan, others

Drugs That Reduce Stickiness of Blood Platelets (Not Blood Thinners)

Acetylsalicylic acid	Aspirin, enteric coated aspirin: Entrophen, Novasen
Dipyridamole	Persantin, Persantine
Potassium supplements (see Tabel 5)	

DRUGS THAT REDUCE CHOLESTEROL

Fibrates

Bezafibrate	Bezalip, Bezalip-Mono
Gemfibrozil	Lopid
Fenofibrate	Lipidil, Lipidil-Micro

Resins

Cholestyramine	Questran
Colestipol	Colestid

Statins

Fluvastatin	Lescol
Lovastatin	Mevacor
Pravastatin	Pravachol
Simvastatin	Zocor

Appendix B

NORMAL VALUES OR NORMAL RANGE
OF SOME BLOOD CONSTITUENTS

---

mg/dL = milligram per 100 ml of blood
mEq/L = milliequivalent per liter of blood
mmol/L = millimole per liter of blood

	United States		Canada, U.K. (S.I.)
Cholesterol	150 to 200 mg/dL	÷ 40 =	3.7 to 5 mmol/L
HDL cholesterol	40 to 80 mg/dL	÷ 40 =	1 to 2 mmol/L:
LDL cholesterol	60 to 160 mg/dl	÷ 40 =	1.5 to 4 mmol/L
LDL cholesterol (optimal)	less than 130 mg/dL	÷ 40 =	less than 3.3 mmol/L
LDL cholesterol (if heart trouble)	less than 100 mg/dL	÷ 40 =	less than 2.6 mmol/L
Creatinine (test of kidney function)	less than 1.4 mg/dL		less than 130 µmol/L
Potassium	4 to 5 mEq/L		4 to 5 mmol/L
Triglycerides	50 to 300 mg/dL	÷ 100 =	0.5 to 3 mmol/L